CONQUER THE BAR

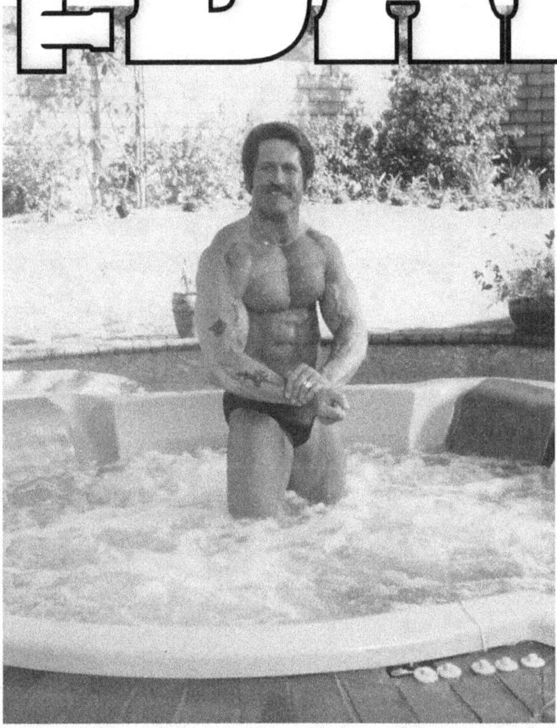

(The Real Rocky Unplugged)

story written by John D. Motta

from acquired tapes of Rocky's life story

ISBN: 1467959812
ISBN-13: 9781467959810

DEDICATION

IN HONOR OF ROCKY:
Whose spirit and love for the Lord remain today,
we are blessed to share his incredible story with you.

A special thanks to Rocky and Trudy's blended family of 3
wonderful daughters Sally, Jody, and Jennifer. We want to
personally thank them for the 5 'challenging' grandchildren who
have been a source of love and enjoyment throughout the years.

To all the prayer warriors especially Melissa, Ingrid, Linda, Joan,
and Juanita who have never left my side. I thank you, God bless.

Trudy

Dedicated to the three precious loves of my life Katie, Cassie,
and Kara who faithfully support my love of the written word. I'm
so very proud of the talented young ladies you have become…
just remember, you are never too old to call me 'Daddy'!

John

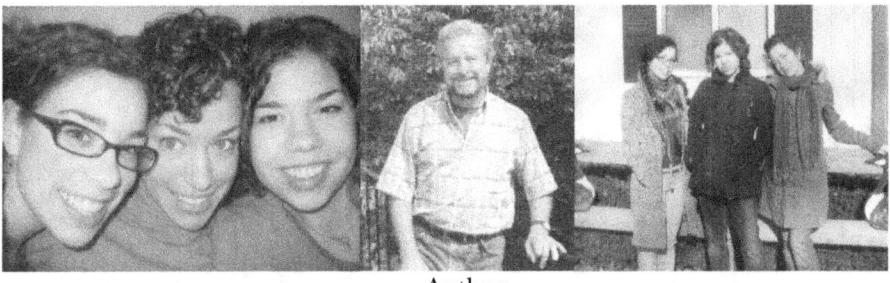

Kara, Cassie, and Katie

Author
John Dean Motta

ROCKY'S RIDE
Prologue

Norman "Rocky" Rauch staved off fatal cancer not once but three times.

In his glory days, Rocky had been a man of superhuman strength. He qualified in Denver, Colorado, to represent the United States in weightlifting at the 1964 Olympic Games. It was prior to the Olympics in Minneapolis, Minnesota, during participation in the North American Championships, that the Olympic candidate hyperextended an elbow, severely tearing the muscle in his forearm. Refusing to accept defeat, Rocky remarkably returned to the training room and applied some ointment to the torn muscle while wrapping his elbow in an Ace bandage. Then he returned to the competition to power clean and jerk 300 pounds, winning the heavyweight division against all odds. But this freak injury had axed his dreams of competing for the coveted gold medal in the upcoming 1964 Olympics, and years of tedious physical therapy and mental anguish followed.

To most people, sweating and straining for hours on end during workouts was a sacrifice, a drudgery. But training in a gym with barbells was as much a part of Rocky's daily routine as morning doughnuts and coffee were to other people. He excelled in his workout sessions. Rocky broke so many records and collected so many trophies over the years that winning championship competitions became almost mundane.

Later in life Rocky successfully switched careers from Olympic power lifting to bodybuilding, something not many champion lifters could achieve. He conquered this sport as well. In 1983 he was crowned Mr. America Over 40 in the premiere bodybuilding championship for men past their prime. Norman Rauch's physical accomplishments on a national level in weightlifting and bodybuilding are mind-boggling and, in his case, death-defying.

Self-inflicted cancer was the diagnosis of numerous specialists who treated Rocky's cancer. Deep down in the darkest hollow of his eternal soul, Rocky knew better than any of his medical doctors that his many years of self-inflicted anabolic steroid abuse were what nearly cost him his life.

Linda, a young writer who first attempted to compose this incredible "hanging on to life by a thread" story, first met Rocky through fate. As a regional director for a well-known bath company, he was on a business trip attending a whirlpool bath convention in Dallas, Texas. Tracie, Linda's best friend of many years, owned and operated a cappuccino coffee stand in the Dallas Convention Center. Rocky asked for a glass of water with a deep and husky voice, the magnitude matching his grandiose frame. Tracie watched this giant of a man wash down half a hundred vitamins of every conceivable shape and color. When she inquired as to why he was taking such a horse-choking variety of pills, Rocky briefly outlined his history.

Almost in shock, Tracie spoke up once again, "Your life has been incredible! You should write a book." His charismatic and easygoing personality made their dialogue comfortable even though the two had just met.

"Everybody tells me that," stated Rocky. "In fact, a lot of people call me the 'real' Rocky." He snickered. Rocky's battle to win back his life from the dreadful cancer had all but smothered a muscle-bound ego. "But I don't know any writers, and I'm so busy with my job. I just don't know. I've never taken the time to pursue an autobiography."

It was then that Tracie scribbled down Linda's phone number for him. "Linda is a writer. She lives on a horse ranch in Montana. Give her a call."

Rocky made it a priority to give this Linda a call. Before she ever met Norman Rauch in person, she found herself thoroughly impressed with his honesty. He told her that he took full responsibility for damaging his own health, admitting freely that his own ego-driven obsession with being a winner caused him to take massive doses of steroids, which was plainly and simply the wrong thing to do. This is something that Rocky knew he had to live with and pay the consequences for. He liked to speak to as many young people as he could line up in high school assembly halls. Mr. Rauch talked about the stupidity of going for the "quick fix" of building a brawny frame through the use of anabolic steroids. "Take it from a guy who's been there: muscles aren't worth dying over."

It was Rocky's courage that impressed Linda the most. His last battle with cancer required a full bone marrow transplant, which kept him immobilized for fifty-nine days. He experienced numerous unforeseen complications that nearly killed him throughout the transplant process, yet his extraordinary mental courage and physical discipline, his determination to "train for living" once his cancer was diagnosed and his loving relationship with his wife Trudy saw him through the torturous procedures. After his bone marrow transplant, Rocky went on to win a medal in the 1991 World Transplant Olympics, which were held in Budapest, Hungary.

Linda and her husband raised horses on a ranch outside of Butte, Montana. Their location was at the end of a quiet and serene road, surrounded only by the sounds and sights of elk, deer, horses, and an occasional moose.

Rocky ended his last phone conversation with Linda in his usual customary and positive manner. "Trudy and I will drive out to Montana for a week this summer. We'll get my life story down on tape, ride a few horses, barbeque a few steaks, and have a few laughs. If the book works out, then great! If not, we'll have had a fun vacation out west."

You could hear the love and enthusiasm that Rocky had for his wife in his voice. "Trudy and I could use a break from all the stress and strain going on in our lives. We're both very fond of animals, especially Trudy. She loves to ride horses. In fact, she was a state pole bending champion in high school. I owe her a relaxing trip after all she's had to go through with me and the cancer procedures over the years." Rocky then let out another hearty chuckle over his absurd reasoning. "I can't believe that I just said that. I owe Trudy more than just a vacation. I owe her my life! But it's a place to start."

The following is a factual account of Rocky's life. Steroid rages and his compulsive drive to be deemed the strongest man in the world drove away three wives—nearly four. It took a near- death experience with cancer, a great woman, and a born-again Christian belief in the Father Almighty to get his priorities in order. ROCKY'S ROAD twists and curves, viciously in some sections and triumphantly in others. As Rocky says, "My life has truly been a rocky ride."

This prologue was taken from the memoirs of Linda Yeagle, who made an excellent effort to write the life story of Norman "Rocky" Rauch. For one reason or another, the book was never completed at that time, but Norman Rauch was granted permission to use Linda's personal accounts.

CHAPTER 1
MOVING TO WHERE
THE PASTURE GETS GREENER

As the dust was settling from the massive cloudburst of earthy particles, a large silhouette viewed the double plow-horse disc vanish over the horizon. A young man of ten years old was trying to see how many jagged rocks he could blast through the space just under the barbed wire fence. He was big and muscular for his age. The boy had dreams of becoming a sports figure as soon as he was old enough.

The distant, bright-orange ball of light was just starting to hover over the MARK'S FARM front gate sign in the western sky. It would be getting dark soon, and it was time for the young man to head back down the beaten path for the homestead.

The young man's father, Henry Steven Rauch, was a very strict, stern man. He meant well but was not always a loving or hugging type of a person. He was a plumber by trade, belonging to the local plumber's union. According to the record books, he almost never took a day off for being ill. His family had never taken a vacation together. Henry Steven always proclaimed that he wanted to get his hands on every cent he could to support the family. The slender but strong ten-year-old threw one more circular rock and smacked it with his baseball bat. He watched it soar over the bullpen center fence. "That one was for the Gipper!" exclaimed Norman.

As the young boy was walking back home from Farmer Mark's surrounding fence, he could see a sign in his second-story home window that read: FOR SALE BY OWNER. He had heard his mother and father converse about moving a couple of times but had never given it much thought until now. The sign must have been hung after Henry Steven came home from his work. The rural farm life was like heaven to Henry Steven's young son. The boy did not want to leave his life of country freedom.

As the young man walked through the swinging back porch door, his mother Dorothy said in a raging voice, "Norman, you're late for supper. Sit down before your biscuits with my special-flavored gravy get cold." Dorothy Irene's heritage was Pennsylvanian Dutch. She came from a large peace-spoken family. Her son Norman always thought of his mother as too much of a perfectionist.

"Hey, Pops, what's up with that FOR SALE sign in the upstairs spare room window?" spoke Norman in a heavier-than-usual tone of voice.

"What do you mean what's up with that sign?" asked his father Henry. "Is that how you kids talk today? It's *up* in the upstairs window. You know how your mother and I have been talking about moving into the city for some time now. You never know how the union's going to treat you. One day there's more work than you can possibly handle. The next day there could be none."

Norman Rauch was born on March 11, 1942, in the Allentown, Pennsylvania, hospital. When he was around five years of age, Norman used to romp around his grandmother's living room, usually dressed in his sun suit and wearing his cute little brown-and-white shoes. Even though he was big for his age, Norman was sometimes mistaken for a girl. He had long, blonde, curly locks of hair that made him look as cute as a button—or that's what his grandmother, Sally Hoffman, used to brag about, anyway. Norman would sometimes rock in his grandmother's rocking chair while watching her hand-knit white doilies on the sofa bed near her marble coffee table. Grandma Hoffman spoiled her grandson every chance she got.

Then one day Norman's mother cut his long beautiful locks of shiny golden hair. But Norman didn't mind. He thought it was cool, as in there was no air-conditioning back in the 1940s. Norman even used to strip off his clothes sometimes and lie naked, face-down on the marble coffee table. It kept his soft baby skin cool and comfortable. Grandmother Hoffman lived in a row house that consisted of ten to twelve living quarters all connected together. There was a dividing wall for every two houses. It was said that if you knocked hard enough on your connecting wall, your neighbors would hear you at the corners. Aunt Florence, the "old maid" of the family, also lived with Nanna and spoiled Norman.

Ten years after Norman's birth, the immediate family packed all of their belongings and moved into the heart of Allentown. As the weeks went by, Henry Steven would arrive home after work later and later every night. At first it was only once in a while. One summer night during the middle of the week, Dorothy Irene had her husband's favorite meal all ready to be served with the table set at 4:55 p.m. The family had always eaten supper exactly at 5:00 p.m. back on the farm unless Henry had to work overtime.

"Your father might not be very happy with my decision, son," expressed Dorothy, "but go ahead and start cutting your steak. I'll pour you a glass of lemonade. Growing boys need their nourishment. I don't know where your father could possibly be. He never called to say he had to work late."

"Maybe Pops had to help one of his buddies move or something," Norman suggested. "You know how he's always trying to help people."

"I know, dear," said his mother. "I'll just call and if I can get that new operator to patch me through." The first call was made to the CORNER TAP on Broadway and Fifth Street. "Hello. Is Henry Rauch there, by chance? Perhaps I could speak to him if he is."

"Nobody here by that name, madam," said the man on the phone. Click.

"Where could that man of mine be?" thought Dorothy.

A couple of hours later Henry stumbled into the living room with a fellow companion. "Hey, where's my sup...supper at, Ma?" Henry asked, also stumbling with his speech. "I brought my good old pal Joe home with me, 'cause he's star...starving too. Then we're going to go out and get us a couple dozen of those damn night crawlers for some night fishing. I just bought Joe's old boat, and I've got to make sure it doesn't sink before I pay him in full. Where's the boy? How come he's not at the supper table? That kid better not be getting in trouble somewhere."

"Sit down, Henry. You're drunk," said Dorothy. "I will bring you your supper this time, and I'll also put a pot on the stove burner for coffee. Me and the boy already ate your favorite supper. You two can have the leftovers from yesterday."

Henry was, for the most part, a good person when he was sober. But when he came home from a binge, Henry could be spiteful and bitter. He did take his son out fishing a few times in that old rowboat. When Norman turned 15 years of age, his father bought him a 410 shotgun for his birthday. Henry Steven taught his son the proper techniques for hunting deer and trapping bear.

"I am very grateful that I was able to take off a little early tonight and celebrate Uncle Sam's birthday with my favorite people in the entire world!" exclaimed Henry Steven.

"Slow down a bit, Henry," insisted Dorothy. "The night's still young. Let's savor this moment. This is a great country. We should appreciate that we have each other and our wonderful son, Norman."

"You're absolutely right, my dear," agreed Henry. "But let's savor a couple more imported beers."

"Coming right up, Mr. Rauch," said the maître d'. "Also, the special for this evening is a seasoned matelote stewed to your taste, sir."

"And what exactly is that special?" asked Dorothy.

"This specialty is a stew of fish in a fine wine and oil, madam," quoted the fancy head waiter. "I'll be right back with your drinks."

"What did that funny looking little waiter just say, Ma?" asked Norman.

"Oh, here it is on the menu," said Dorothy. "It is a stew of a certain type of fish in wine and oil. That maître d' was absolutely correct. Give him a large tip at the end of the night, Henry."

"Well, since we are at a clam bake tonight, I think I'll go with fish instead of steak," said Henry Steven. After the main course Henry ordered another round of beverages for himself, Dorothy, and the table of adults sitting next to them. They were all seated in the back section of the exterior porch deck near the side entrance-way arbor. You could actually view the seafood being prepared from that angle. The canopy overhead protected the enormous crowd from the elements.

After finishing his last bite of pie a la mode, Norman said, "Thanks Pops and Mama for the delicious meal, but I'm starting to feel chilly, and it's getting dark. Remember there's a special episode of *Sing Along with Mitch* on at 9:00 tonight. Can we please get going soon?"

"Just hold your horses there, son," answered Henry Steven. "Me and your Ma are just starting to have some fun. If you're going to wimp out on us, then go sit in the truck. There's even an old sleeping bag in the back."

Just before Norman turned 16 years of age, he thought about what a pleasure it would be to take his Grandmother Sally Hoffman out for a drive in the country. Maybe they could even go back and visit the old stomping grounds. Norman thought it would be a thrill to spoil his grandmother for a change, but first he had to be able to pass his driver's license examination. It was difficult to practice driving during the severe winter conditions of 1958.

One afternoon when Norman entered the kitchen after school, his mother had a tear in her eye. "Honey, I have something to tell you that you're not going to like hearing. Sit down on the couch, dear. Your grandmother passed away this morning."

"What do you mean, Mom?" inquired Norman. "Grandma passed away?"

"Your grandma died early, at the crack of dawn," said Norman's mother. The boy gave his mother a hard cold stare. The sudden news did not penetrate his brain so fast. "But I'm sure she's up in heaven right now as we—"

"No!" interrupted the boy. "Grandma can't be gone. I'm going to get my driver's license in a couple of weeks, and I'm supposed to pick her up in Quaker Town. I wanted to drive her back to the farm." Norman was full of anger that was rushing out like a jail convict attempting an escape. "Why Grandma Sally? Why my grandmother, Lord? Why didn't you take me instead? She didn't hurt anybody, and she always prayed to you. And I always thought of you as my big Gipper. I don't really like you anymore." Norman was hysterical for some time. He loved his grandmother dearly.

Aunt Florence walked over and sat next to her nephew at the wake gathering and said, "My dear Norman, I'm sure you're still too young to even know what death is all about. We all came from ashes and will return to ashes. Your grandmother is watching over us right at this very moment. It was meant to be, son. God called upon her—"

"Yeah, but I didn't get a chance to fulfill one of my dreams," Norman told his Aunt Florence. "I wanted to show her how good of a driver I'm going to be."

"She is still very proud of you from where she's at now," said Aunt Florence. "Now to cheer us both up a little, I would like to tell you a story. Your father Henry was living on Adam's Island before you were even a twinkle in your mother's eye. He had side gigs on weekends driving his band member buddies around in his limousine. You see, son, it was the Big Band Era with Tiny Hill and the King of Swing."

"What are gigs?" asked Norman.

"Gigs were the band jobs that your father worked at, carrying the equipment and setting up instruments," answered Florence.

"How do you know all about my father's life before I was born?" asked Norman, a bit inquisitive.

"I know all about Henry Steven because I used to date him before your mother came into the picture," smirked Florence. "We only dated a couple of times because your father thought that I was too bossy. But you know what? I thought your father was stubborn like a big rock! You couldn't get him to budge for nothing if he didn't want to. A few of his buddies used to call him Rock—the ones who didn't call him Whitey 'cause of his bleached blonde hair."

"I love nicknames!" exclaimed young Norman. "I wish people would call me something other than Rauschie."

"And that is the way the Pennsylvanian Dutch people pronounce your last name, Norman," interrupted Aunt Florence. "Rouk."

"Just call me Tiger," chuckled Norman. "Do you think that Grandma Hoffman up in heaven will approve?"

"She will, but I don't think that your mother will," explained Florence. "And it's hard to tell about your father."

"Tell me more about my parents, Aunt Florence," said Norman. "You're starting to cheer me up a little."

"All right. A long time ago there was a gentleman by the name of Barry Reed, who was in that Glen Miller type of band that I was telling you about," Florence said. "Well, your father used to drive Mr. Reed and the other band members to their engagements. One weekend night before one of those big band gigs, your father drove over to your mother's house to pick her up. We were all going on a double date.

"Your father Henry walked into your mother's house at the time and saw her playing her upright acoustic piano as he entered through the front doorway. Then he noticed a photograph of her that was vibrating on top of the keyboard as your mom played the melody. It was a side view of Dorothy Irene's high school graduation picture. Your father said sarcastically, 'That picture of you on top of the piano was photographed wrong. The photographer must not have known what he was doing. You never take a side view picture of someone with a long schnozzle.'"

"That was cruel of my dad," said Norman. "Some of the kids at school say that I have a large nose. Not to my schnoz, of course."

"Now you're starting to make me feel better," snickered Florence. "I'll tell you a little more about your father before the priest comes out to deliver the eulogy. Whitey played football with the West End Tigers, which was actually in a semi-pro league. He was very fast and competitive. Your father always needed a good challenge. Whitey was always very athletic in his younger days and had many medals and ribbons to prove it. He also couldn't say no to anybody and had a good heart when it came to giving people a hand."

"Why did my father change so much, Aunt Florence?" asked Norman.

"What do you mean, son?" Florence answered with a question.

"Well, you said that Pops—or Whitey, as he was called—was a generous, good-hearted man," stated Norman. "I sometimes don't believe that he treats me or Mom with much respect. Once I got into a little bit of trouble at school with a teacher. He said that I sarcastically talked out of turn without raising my hand. When Pops found out from Mom that night after coming home late for supper, he wouldn't even talk things out with her. Instead he drug me down into the wine cellar and whacked me a couple of times on the hind end with his leather belt."

"I hate to say this, but your father might have been a bit snookered up on alcohol that evening," explained Aunt Florence.

"I don't like it when people drink," said Norm. "Grandma Hoffman read bible passages to me when I was younger. She often said that humans do strange things sometimes when they take a few too many nips of that firewater. Sometimes even great leaders from the bible would get themselves in trouble from that unpredictable fermented grape juice."

After Sally Hoffman's wake was over and everyone gave their condolences, Norm still looked somewhat peckish to his mother. "Come on, son," said Dorothy. "It's time that we all went home and got some rest."

"But Mother, Aunt Florence said that she'd drive me home," answered the boy. "We might even stop off for a double-malted shake." Norm wanted to get another small burden off of his chest.

At the ice cream parlor, Norman did one complete spin on the circular mounted seat and grinned at his aunt. Florence in turn tried the same spin on her counter seat and said, "That just made my head spin! Isn't this fun?" Since it was too cold for car hops, the two "kids" had fun spanning the polka dotted wall décor with their stares. "Now what was it that you wanted to tell me?"

"Well, I'll start from the beginning," Norm began. "When I was around seven, I heard about the circus coming to town. It was every kid's dream: to go and watch the circus people put up the Big Top. I can still picture the ringmaster with the stove pipe top hat shouting, 'The one and only high wire act that's never been performed before in front of an audience is about ready to begin. Focus your eyes toward the peak of the Big Top tent!' I've never confessed this to anybody until now. I actually stole my mom's silver dollar collection out of her forbidden drawer to get into the sideshows at the circus. I walked five or six miles to get to the Allentown fairgrounds, and I had a great time that afternoon.

"My father had to come home early and go down to the fairgrounds to look for me, and he did not look too thrilled when he spotted me talking to a bearded lady. As you can probably imagine, I got the tar beat out of me when we arrived back home, and I don't believe that Pops was liquored up. I know now that I was wrong for stealing those shiny silver dollars, but back then it was well worth it just to see eighteen clowns fit into a Studebaker jalopy."

As the waitress grabbed the steel milk shake container off of the industrial strength Mixmaster, she said, "That was one double-malted chocolate shake for the boy and one large double black cow for you, ma'am. Coming right up. Here's your ticket. That'll be a total of $1.10 plus tax. Pay at the register on the way out. Now does anyone need a refill or anything at the counter before I take my smoke break?"

"Aunt Florence, wasn't it you and Grandma Hoffman who bought me that pet bunny and those colored peepies that one Easter around 1949?" asked Norman.

"Yes, I remember," said Aunt Florence as she sipped her root beer float through a straw. "What ever happened to that pet jackrabbit?"

"I was just about ready to get to that," explained Norm. "Well, my father actually went through the roof at first. He had to build a rabbit pen and a shelter for the baby chicks to keep them all contained. When my pet bunny grew to about the size of a small moose, Pops said that it had outgrown its welcome and that it was time for it to go. I'll never forget watching my father butcher my pet bunny rabbit for the supper table. Mother actually broiled my rabbit one day and set it right next to my father's plate. She and I watched Pops pick all of the medium-well baked meat off the skeleton like a carnivorous mammal. We didn't have the heart to touch that once-a-floppy-eared rabbit. I remember going to my room and crying myself to sleep."

"That's a crying shame," said Florence, "but you are growing up now and becoming a young man. I'm just happy that you are getting all of these things out of your system. Maybe you should put all of this behind you and work on your future. Let me hear about what kind of athlete you want to be when you grow another six inches?"

"Bear with me for one more chicken shit story," snickered Norm. "Then I'll tell you what I have planned for my future."

"Well, I guess you are growing older," chuckled Aunt Florence, "you already know how to say the S-word. So how many more stories you got left in you? We might have to go for two more doubles. And I'm not talking baseball either."

"I remember raising chickens a while back," stated Norm. "Actually, my father built the chicken pen, and my parents raised them. I used to torment them! Remember I was young and spunky and didn't know what I was doing. Anyway, one late afternoon I was pushing a long pointed stick through the chicken wire fence to tease the chicken hens. Then I got a brainstorm for a kid of around five. I whipped out my pee shooter and sprayed one of the roosters right on the comb with my circulating waterfall. What I didn't know was that my father was watching me all this time from the upstairs bathroom window.

"With just a towel wrapped around his lower body he yelled out at me to leave the chickens alone or he was going to come down and tan my hide. Still to this moment I don't remember what I said to him. My father actually laughed when he told me about this experience not more than two years ago. I guess I didn't believe that he would prance through the backyard jungle wearing just a small towel that could fall off at any moment. Well, he did come after me. When Pops caught up with me he picked me up by the ankles, turned me upside down, and beat me to a pulp."

"I should be driving both of us home soon," stated Aunt Florence, "before I get into trouble with your parents."

"Yeah, I'm getting a little sleepy now," said Norm as he put his hand to his mouth and yawned.

"I'll give you a break this time," explained Norm's aunt. "I'll let you tell me all about your future goals next time we meet."

As the young man reached his untidy bedroom, he let his clothes fall into a heap on the hardwood floor and fell into a deep slumber.

As he was rounding the stuffed gunny sack bases, he pictured himself just slamming a towering fly ball over the center field fence in Forbes Field. Even the Say Hey Kid couldn't reach that one to make another one of his incredible basket catches. As Norm reached home plate he looked up into the heavens and saw the light of a bright white angel with silver wings and a golden halo looking down upon him. "That one was definitely for my father, Whitey Rauch," bragged Norm. That walk-off homerun won the game in the twelfth inning by the score of the Pittsburg Pirates 2 and the New York Giants 1.

All of a sudden Norm found himself staring down a narrow white chalk line at a partially-built rectangular wooden box. As he sprinted away from the starting blocks into the wind, he could feel a difference in the weight of the long cylindrical pole that he was carrying in the horizontal position. The style of the pole seemed different in touch from the bamboo pole that he was used to. As the momentum of Norm's body, along with the velocity of the lighter fiberglass pole, struck the wooden base box, the young athlete found himself climbing higher and higher into the vault of heaven. "I'm going for the GOLD!" he yelled.

When Norm descended back down from the clouds, a bright red-and-white FOR SALE BY OWNER sign flashing in the old two-story farm house window caught his attention. He always thought of the old "ice house" apartment building that his parents used to rent by Mark's farm as his own two-story castle. "I don't want to move. This farm land is my home!" A large bail of straw broke the boy's fall on the other side of the spider-webbed fence.

Norman woke up in a cold sweat. "Let's come back to reality, Norman," shouted his mother. "It's time to get up and start your chores." Norm's mother had to pull her son by the ankles to force him out of bed. "Come on, son. I have a list of things for you to do. Let's go. Skedaddle!"

The boy staggered into the kitchen and reached up to grab a box of Frosted Flakes out of the cupboard. Then he walked over and turned on the old black-and-white Bendix television set. Norm sat down on the sofa bed in his boxer shorts and said, "Hey, Ma, when are we going to get another TV? This one's on the blink again. I think we need another pair of rabbit ears. *Garfield Goose* starts in fifteen minutes."

"You surely liked it back in 1949 when it was the very first television set on the block," said Dorothy Irene. "All your school friends were here every night after school. Now come on, Norman. Put your cereal in a bowl like normal kids, and then go get dressed and start your chores." Norm's mother handed him a list with four or five things to do before he got to go out and play with his buddies.

It took the boy approximately twenty minutes to make his bed, fifteen minutes to throw all his stuff in the closet, and forty minutes to pick up all his dirty laundry and finish one washtub load. "Can I get going now, please?" asked Norm.

"Now how do you ask me that again?" asked Dorothy.

Norm gave his mother a strange look and then looked around the room and said, "All right, Ma, but you know I'm getting too old to talk like this. May I get going to meet my buddies, pretty please with sugar on top?"

"You may go after you start one more load of your smelly undershirts and socks," said Dorothy Irene. "I'll work out the grass stains from your overalls on the washboard. And don't carry any matches with you. You remember what you did at the old apartment in Mrs. Fry's clothesline porch area, don't you?"

"Mom, I'm trying to forget about those bad moments when I was young and stupid," explained Norm. "I was only doing what every kid does before they grow up."

"I'll never forget the look on Mrs. Fry's face when she saw all of her nightgowns and undergarments going up in smoke," chuckled Dorothy. "I thought she was going to croak from a heart attack."

"I'm leaving now, Mother," stated Norm. "Oh, and by the way, call me Tiger from now on."

CHAPTER 2
THE REAL WORLD

The last couple of drops of wet white flakes splashed across the windshield of the Baringer Bakery delivery truck as it pulled away from the curb for the next stop. There were snow drifts as deep as fourteen inches on some of the side streets of downtown Allentown. The sun was just starting to become visible. The next delivery location was a restaurant that hadn't opened its doors to the public yet, so the delivery driver sloshed through the wet drifting snow and placed five boxes of doughnuts in the entranceway and was off again on his route.

"Wake up, son," yelled Henry Steven. "I'm telling you for the second and last time to get your tired ass out of bed. It's 5:23 a.m. and you need to get going to keep your customers satisfied." Norm worked for the MORNING CALL newspaper as a delivery boy and collector of bills that were due or past due. This was a real-life challenge. He was getting his first taste of the sales life in the real world. Not everyone would pay for their subscription on time. Some people were dishonest and would try to stiff the boy. People had excuses for everything.

Half-awake, Norm stuffed the inserts into the Saturday morning edition of the MORNING CALL. He then strapped his four-and-a-half bundles of papers onto his snow runner sled and took off by pulling it down the uncleared snowy trail. This was his second year on the route. As a freshman, he was mesmerized by the thought of becoming an Olympic bodybuilder someday, so he worked very hard to earn money to help pay for extra food and supplies. All he could think about was going over to his friend's house later on to bulk up with heavy iron weights. In order to build up that physique, he needed quite a lot of protein. At the time he was a little on the pudgy side and was trying not to consume double helpings of everything at the supper table.

Norm was running about forty-five minutes late because of the fresh wet snow. Because he was behind schedule now, he had to deal with the real world. As he flung a perfectly folded paper up on his fifth customer's porch, an elderly man in his shiny silk bath robe yelled out, "You'd better get my paper here on time! You're an hour late!"

"It's a rough ride plowing through all this slush," Norm shouted back, challenging the older customer. "By the way, sir, would you care to receive a Christmas calendar compliments of the MORN-ING CALL? They're free!"

"Now what would I do with a calendar, boy? I'm retired!" yelled the customer right back. "I don't need to know about times and dates and holidays and stuff. The only thing I care about is when my morning paper arrives late!"

"I'll try to have it here on time tomorrow, mister," said Norm apologetically. Then he added under his breath, "You old' goat. I'll be back at the end of next week to collect for this month's bill."

"Remember, boy, only come around to get your money when the missus is here," chuckled the customer. "She wears the pants in the family, and I wear the smoking jacket."

Norm ignored the old man's comments and let his thoughts wander. He had more important things to think about. To build a physique with a barrel chest and a washboard stomach was his dream. "I need to bulk up on more protein and carbohydrates," he thought.

Large multi-patterned white snowflakes were falling from the heavens once again. Norm finally made it to one of the local eatery establishments and ducked into the front entrance and out of the uncontrollable weather. Much to his surprise, he practically tripped over a pile of assorted doughnuts. It was still very early, and nobody was around yet, so he helped himself to about a half-dozen jam– and lemon-filled pastries. He shoved four into his side coat pockets while shoveling two down his throat. A strong belch was let loose, and it was time for him to fly. Now he was in desperate need to find a thirst quencher.

The double blades on the wooden sled made a wide turn while etching a rail pattern through the slushy, compacted flakes. Another bundle of folded papers was snatched from the sled before it was concealed under the rear porch deck of the attached business buildings. Norman climbed three flights of stairs while flinging the folded papers against the back doors of the various proprietary shops and upstairs apartments.

All of a sudden he noticed the name "Lehigh Valley Dairy" inscribed on a decrepit wooden milk container. It was full of hourglass-shaped bottles with the upper circular compartment filled with fresh, rich cream. The boy lifted a couple of the bottles out of the milk container and spotted a row of cardboard waxed boxes full of what appeared to be chocolate milk. Then he lifted a quart box up about chest high. "Just what the doctor ordered," he said under his breath.

He chugged the quart box of chocolate milk to quench his thirst. There was protein in the milk. He'd read about it on the ingredient label. A voice entered his mind: "Go ahead and down another one. Milk's good for building up your muscles." Norm knew that he had the money to pay for the milk and doughnuts, but he received a tingling sensation in the spinal column every time he acknowledged a challenge like this. It was sort of a thrill to be on the devil's side of the court. So he snitched another box of chocolate milk and was on his way, even though Norm knew stealing was wrong according to one of God's Ten Commandments.

The following Friday night he was back out in action once again on the MORNING CALL route. This time he was trying to kill two birds with one stone. The customers were very willing to receive their bundle of news but were sometimes hesitant when it came to paying on time. One stop at a local restaurant turned out to be somewhat distasteful.

"How you doing there, son?" asked the proprietor. "I just have to ask you one question before I pay you for what my total bill comes to."

"Yes, sir," hesitated Norman.

"Have you seen anyone stealing doughnuts out of the boxes at the front entrance on the weekend mornings?" asked the restaurant owner.

"No, sir," stated the boy, "but I'll let you know if I do."

"Well, I guess I'll pay you this time for your service, son," said the proprietor. "But I will catch the thief who's taking a bite out of my profits red-handed if it takes me the rest of the week!" Norman accepted the money he had coming to him, gave the business owner 20 cents from a $2.00 bill, and quickly got the hell out of there.

Norm made a painful mistake by returning to the scene of the crime on the following Sunday morning. He went for two more doughnuts and stuffed them into his coat pockets once again. Before school on Monday morning, Norman wolfed down the two doughnuts with a glass of white milk from home. After being at school for only a short time he raised his hand and asked the teacher to use the bathroom. He was dismissed a total of three times. The third time he went to get an excuse from the school nurse to go home. The thought of ever eating another doughnut again in his lifetime made the boy want to throw away his mother's subscription to the magazine *Roll Your Own Batter*. His stomach turned so many times that he just stayed there on the pot with his elbows on his knees and his hands keeping his head from crashing onto the floor.

The next time he swung by the local Eatery Restaurant to deliver the newspaper, the owner was waiting at the door entrance, "The cross-town bakery was delighted by my orders to mix in a certain amount of ex-lax into the doughnut batter. That doughnut thief must have been crapping his brains out for a couple of days straight!"

"I wonder if he knew it was me all along," thought Norman.

You could sniff the sweet odor of the fresh cut grass clippings from the neighbor's lawn. It was summertime once again, and

Norman was off and running. The fairgrounds were open, and some of his friends were tagging along. They had heard that there was a tattoo tent open for business. The movie *The Rose* was playing at the outdoor theatre, and Norm just had to have a tattoo of a rose inscribed on his body. The cost of a tattoo of that caliber was $2.50. He always carried large amounts of change that he had earned from his newspaper collection in his baggy pants pockets. Two weeks later, the boys went to a cross-town tattoo parlor, and Norm had to get the "snakehead with a dagger through it" tattoo that was at a special discounted price.

In the middle of July Dorothy Irene could not figure out why her son was always prancing around with long-sleeved shirts on. "Come here a minute, son," said Dorothy. "What are all these dark red stains on your shirts from?"

"Oh, that's nothing," explained Norman. "I'm still doing forearm blocks with my friends. I want to at least make the third or maybe even the second string roster on the football team next year. That could be dried blood from a scratch from one of us, Ma." Norm continued to hide his bleeding tattoos from his parents. He knew that his father would kill him if he ever found out.

His dad was a good football player and took it seriously, and Norman wanted to somehow make his father proud of him. He had been cut from the third string junior varsity team last season. The thought of making father proud made Norm strive that much harder by practicing over the summer. Nothing ever came as easy for him as it did for some of his classmates. One of them, Bobby Becker, had the gift of playing football and the instinct of being great, and naturally, he acquired the cockiness that goes along with it.

Norman could not hide his tattoos forever. When Henry Steven finally found out, he was simply furious. Aunt Althia said that she would pay to have the tattoos surgically removed by a plastic surgeon until she was astounded by the initial cost.

Norman was flexing his biceps in the hallway mirror just after he brushed his teeth with the new Ipana toothpaste that his mother just bought. He thought that he had remembered seeing an eager beaver brushing his teeth in a black-and-white Ipana commercial just the other day. It was a cool, breezy Friday night in October, and Norman was all set to go out to the YWCA youth dance. He had just collected some change from some of his paper route customers and put his percentage into both his front pockets where he could feel it.

After arriving at the dance with his four buddies, Norm drifted in through the front door, leading the pack. The song lyrics, "Every night at ten we do it again," were playing over the loud speaker system. After standing around with his friends for a couple of songs, he decided to go out into the hallway by himself to check something out. All of a sudden Norm caught a glimpse of Bobby Becker moving toward him. Bobby just happened to have someone alongside him who he wanted Norm to meet. It was an ugly, intimidating guy by the name of Barry, who walked right up, got into Norm's face and said, "Give me two bits."

Norman answered, "I don't have two bits."

Then Barry reached down and jingled Norman's left pocket, brushing against his family jewels, and said, "Give me two bits."

Looking a little nervous now, the entrapped boy said once again, "I don't have two bits to give you, pizza face." Barry hauled off and smacked Norm directly across the face, which made his cheek and eye swell up immediately. He tried to brace himself because he saw the punch coming, but that just made things worse. He was hit with a sucker punch from behind by the fist of Bobby Becker. He had a large class ring on at the time and cracked Norm's jaw in two places. The two bullies left him stranded there and ran off. To Norman and his peers, Becker was classified as a chicken shithead. But to Becker's boys, he was known as One-Punch Becker after that.

A couple of his companions helped Norman to get back up on his feet. "What happened, Norman?" asked a friend. "We can't even leave you out of our sight for more than ten minutes, and look what you got yourself into."

"Those two jokers tried to roll me, but I wouldn't give in!" exclaimed Norman. "They aren't getting a nickel from me!" His buddies gave him a lift home. He had a hard time falling asleep that night, mainly because of the pain, but partially because of being afraid of what his dad was going to say to him.

The next morning Norman entered the kitchen, where his father was looking through the sports section of the MORNING CALL. He did not want his dad to notice him, so he reached for a bowl and a box of cereal out of the cupboard. Norman turned around, and Henry Steven was staring straight at his face. "What happened, boy? Somebody really get the best of you?" Norman tried to answer his father but couldn't. He attempted to speak but could not move his jaw.

Henry Steven jumped up from the breakfast table, reached for the telephone on the wall, and gave it three cranks. "Operator, patch me in to the doctor's office up the street," demanded Henry Steven. "My boy needs attention immediately. Tell the nurse on duty that this is an emergency." Norman was sent to the local practitioner's office, which was located about half a block away. His father followed about ten minutes behind after making another phone call.

Father and son waited in a crowded room of patients for the doctor to come out for them. Norm was briefly analyzed and then told that he would have to go to the Allentown Hospital immediately for x-rays. They didn't have that type of equipment in the local doctor's office.

It seemed to Norman that they were never going to stop taking x-rays of his skull. He was later diagnosed with a double fractured jawbone. He needed to be prepared for surgery so the jaw could be wired closed the following morning. Dorothy Irene was notified of her son's condition, and Henry drove straight home to pick her up for an overnight stay.

Bright and early the next morning Norman's jaws were surgically reconstructed. He was under a local anesthetic but was awake to watch his own surgery being performed. His mouth had to be wired shut for two months, and he could only take in liquids with a straw. For a boy who weighed 135 pounds at five foot eleven inches and wanted to play football, this was not an ideal situation, to say the least. Norm had to watch his parents, aunts, and uncles devour turkey and all of the trimmings at Thanksgiving time. He just slurped a cup of eggnog through a straw without giving a hoot about using the proper table manners. Instead of putting on weight for football, he started to look pretty scrawny by Christmastime.

Norman had abundant time to read and think while his jaws were wired shut for that two-month period. One afternoon he purchased a couple of weightlifting magazines with his paper route money. The "built like a rock" physique of Charles Atlas was on the front cover of one of the magazines. "If only I could look like that someday," said Norm to himself. He concentrated on one of the articles about dynamic tension kicks and bodybuilding techniques for some time, holding onto deep feelings that needed to burst out. All he thought about was dynamically kicking the asses of the two mules that had made him suffer.

After the wires were removed and Norm could eat solid foods once again, he tried to find a place to work out. A desk jockey gave him the grand tour of the YMCA basement, where many big shot weightlifters spent a lot of their time. The weight center looked much like a squirrel cage with a giant boiler that was plainly in sight. It had two-by-four-inch framework with chicken wire set up for the walls and steam pipes circulating. There were no windows and no ventilation in that fourteen-by-thirty-foot area, which made it very hot, even in the winter. Norm could picture a bunch of fired-up squirrels pumping iron while roasting their nuts off in front of an open steam pipe.

You were required to be sixteen years of age to lift weights in the luxurious downstairs dungeon. Norman had a feeling that management would figure out his real age of fifteen because he was a member of the main floor swimming pool and recreational area.

The next plan of attack was to check out the Salvation Army where Norm knew Major Hood and went to school with the major's son Neil. This place looked like the better choice of the two workout centers. At the time there were about a half-dozen iron-pumpers exchanging sweat in a twenty-by-twenty-foot converted coal bin.

This was January of 1958. He would be sixteen in a couple of months, so he lied about his age. The scrawny kid of 110 pounds that his peers called Rauschie started his bodybuilding career by pumping iron two hours a day, six days a week. Just reading magazine articles inspired the young man. He knew exactly how he wanted to look when the time was right to take revenge against the enemy.

Norman met a real tough-looking character by the name of Karl Camery. "Call me Buzzard," insisted Karl. "Everyone else does. Nice to meet you, kid." They shook hands, and Karl immediately lay back down on the bench to do another ten repetitions of the bench press. "Spot me, my man," yelled out Karl. "If you want to get somewhere in this world, you have to pay your dues."

As the months passed Buzzard became Norm's trainer and pushed him very hard to meet his goals. He gained approximately ninety pounds from the end of his sophomore year through half of his junior year. Norman listened very closely to the advice of his trainer, and they became tight-bonded friends.

At seventeen Norman was starting to look like a rock. He entered the Teenage Mr. America Contest in 1959, but he didn't place anywhere near the top ten because of all the competition. When he was visiting the YMCA in York, Pennsylvania, the new Norman Rauch was very impressed with the performance of one of the lightweight boys. Dan Sheppard weighed 123 pounds dripping wet and could still press 205 pounds of military weight. He did a standing two-arm press where he cleaned the weight and jerked 205 pounds of wrought iron over his head. Norm was amazed by this kid's ability because he was also pressing around 205 pounds, but he weighed around 200 pounds.

In his senior year in high school, Norman strived as hard as he could to put on another fifty pounds of solid muscle. He was runner-up in the Teenage Nationals that year, and when the Pennsylvania State Weightlifting Championship came around, he was runner-up in that as well.

Norman had started his bodybuilding career for only one important reason: he was bound and determined to gain revenge. Now it was becoming more of a satisfying challenge. He wanted his father to be proud of him for achieving a goal that was getting to be second nature to him. Henry Steven said to him once, "If you get caught at stealing something, cheating on a test, or whatever the case might be, you will pay the consequences. It may take years, but you will get caught in the end. Even cheating your body fits into this category."

Norman was influenced by reading about Yurry Vasloff, a super heavyweight from Russia. In 1960 he could clean and jerk 400 pounds of solid iron. He was two-arm pressing approximately 350 pounds. By reading more and more articles, Norm acquired an inspiration to concentrate heavier on becoming a power weightlifter rather than a bodybuilder.

He read about the three basic types of lifts in competitive weightlifting. The first one that he examined was called the clean and jerk. There were black-and-white photos of weightlifters going through the motions. To clean the weight, the illustration showed a massive weightlifter pulling the weight off of the floor up to his shoulders. Then he immediately jerked the heavy barbell over the head.

The second basic Olympic lift that Norman read about was known as the snatch. The photographs depicted the lift where the bar was grasped and flipped up overhead all in one motion. There were two methods known as the squat or the split style.

The final basic lift mentioned was the two-hand press. The magazine illustrated the Olympic lifter attempting to clean the weight to his shoulders and then suddenly pressing the iron bar straight up over his head.

Norman definitely had the bodybuilding thing down, but he was getting slightly discouraged with his weightlifting attempts. Although Buzzard pushed him very hard in the last two years, the high school senior had no experience with a professional coach. Norm knew that he had to do everything he could because of all the competition out there. He had his work cut out for him.

A few months later the Norm's peers started seeing a drastic improvement in his Olympic lifting ability. Before he graduated from high school, he was cleaning and jerking over 300 pounds, pressing around 250, and snatching more than 230 pounds.

Earlier in his senior year, Norman had showed up for a couple of football practice sessions. The head football coach Jerry Shott had been very impressed with the boy's size. He was the strongest kid on the team. But the coach's philosophy about weightlifting was perfectly clear. One night before the athletes hit the showers, he'd said, "If you guys are going to lift weights, it's going to slow you down. You'll become muscle-bound, your dexterity will be impaired, and you will become very uncoordinated. In other words, you won't even be able to skim a rock across your favorite lake. You'll throw like a girl. You need speed and flexibility to play football on my team!"

Norm had felt that Jerry Shott wasn't going to support him as a football player on the team because of being a weightlifter on the side. When his nose was shattered at one of the next practices, he decided to drop out of the game.

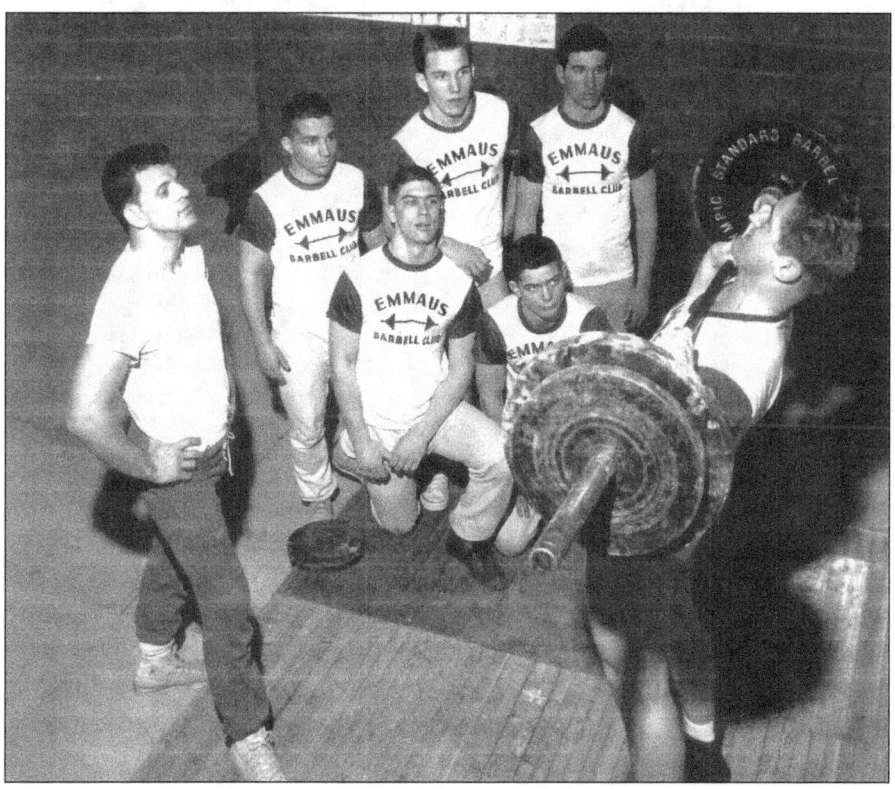

At the Health Club in Emmaus, Pennsylvania, Norm officially cleaned and jerked 300 pounds of solid iron. It just happened to be a very significant date: March 11, 1960. Bob Taffman was the head judge and referee who witnessed that phenomenal feat performed by the young and talented weightlifter. Taffman was like a god to all of the competitors in the business. He knew more about promoting the weightlifting championships than anybody else on the planet. After watching Norman lift, Taffman was amazed and said that he could be the next Olympic champion if he continued his career.

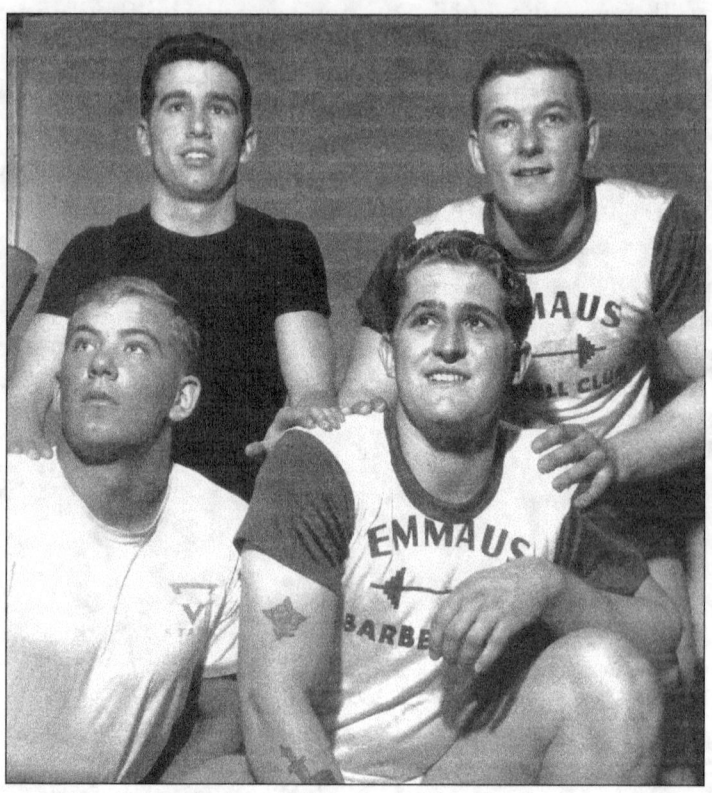

One night after school Norman spotted Bobby Becker on the other side of the street. He had heard that Bobby had quit school because of the upperclassmen teasing him so much. He was still known as "One-Punch Becker." Norman quickly crossed the street, grabbed Becker by the collar, and threw him up against a brick wall. "I should rip your head off!" exclaimed Norman with a stare that almost penetrated the wall.

"Who are you?" asked Bobby Becker, shaking like a leaf on a tree.

"You don't remember when you and Barry Aliverez cracked my jaw in two places?" asked Norm. "I'm Norman Rauch, but you can call me the Rock." Becker's eyes became very wide. The 255-pound kid gave scrawny little Becker a shove. "Get out of my sight." The Becker boy took off running down the street.

Henry Steven and his wife Dorothy had taken legal action against the two renegades after the jaw breaking incident. Barry had a police record a mile long and ended up in a boy's reformatory, a correctional institution that tried to straighten out the lives of young boys before it was too late. Barry was the actual culprit responsible for breaking Norman Rauch's jaw. Bobby Becker received a lighter sentence. He did go back to school but continued to develop a criminal record. Norman's parents gave their son a lot of credit for not physically retaliating against the punk who weighed 130 pounds less than him—except for a couple of shoves and telling the dirt bag that he wasn't worth the trouble.

After school and on weekends Norman took on another job at the Plain and Fancy Diner located across from the football stadium. His job was to clean tables for the waitresses and cut up vegetables for their relish trays. There was also free food involved from a certain list on the menu.

One night after changing into his whites in the downstairs locker room, Norm shuffled up the stairs and into the main kitchen area to report for work when he noticed a brand new dishwasher. It wasn't a machine; it was a person by the name of Barry Aliverez. Norman recognized his ugly mug right off the bat, so he nonchalantly walked up to the creep and growled, "Are you still punching guys out? You still doing two-on-ones?"

"Who are you?" asked Barry.

"I am Norman Rauch," he said. "Remember the guy whose jaw you broke a while back?"

"Holy cow!" exclaimed Barry in amazement. "What did you do to yourself?"

"I built myself up," stated Norman.

"That incident took place a long time ago," explained Barry. "I'm married now and have a two-year-old son. I guess I was sort of wild back then, but I've paid my dues to society, except for you. I would like to apologize for your past disability."

Norman had thought for many months about what he was going to do to this punk if he ever saw him again, and now the time had come. But he remembered one of the lessons his Grandmother Sally Hoffman had taught him about God. The Great Almighty does not want anyone on HIS earth to hold a grudge against any of HIS other children. "You must always learn to turn the other cheek," she would say.

"I'm not going to go that far," thought Norm. "I can't afford to lose any of this hard-earned weight."

Norman let Barry Aliverez off the hook, and the two children of God became good working buddies and best friends for a long time after that.

A couple of nights later Norm was getting some fresh vegetables out of the walk-in cooler when he spotted a huge cherry cheesecake approximately twenty-four inches in diameter. He decided to serve himself a piece when nobody else was looking. Well, one piece led to another and before he knew it, the 255-pound kid had devoured the whole thing. Then he went about his business, making relish trays and wiping up other people's messes. You wouldn't believe what some customers would leave behind.

When he arrived the following scheduled work night, Norman couldn't believe what he saw. The back door had been chained and padlocked shut. There was a sign posted that read: ALL EMPLOYEES ENTER THROUGH THE FRONT DOOR.

"What's this all about?" Norman asked the receptionist at the main entrance.

"You'll find out soon enough," she said with a smirk on her face.

He said to himself, "Well, if they're accusing me, then the most I'll have to do is pay them back for chewing up some of their profits." Norman went straight back to the manager's office to admit to his mistake.

"I know what happened to your cheesecake, if that's what this commotion is all about," explained Norman.

"Did you steal it, boy?" asked Jack, the restaurant manager.

"No, I did not steal it. I ate it."

"You could not have eaten that whole thing," insisted the manager. "Follow me, boy." Jack waddled as fast as his chicken legs could carry him to the walk-in cooler. He briskly grabbed another similar cherry cheesecake, set it down on a stainless steel island in the kitchen, and said, "Show me."

"If I eat this entire cheesecake in your presence," stated Norm, "I would just like to know if I will have to pay for it or the last one."

"If you eat that whole cheesecake right now in front of me," explained the manager, "you will get both free of charge, and you won't be in any kind of trouble."

"Fair enough," said Norman. He had no trouble getting it all down. "You should have believed me, sir. It would have cost you one cake instead of two."

The next day when he went into work there was a sign in the locker room that read, "All employees are only allowed $2.25 a shift for one meal. Anything more than that you'll have to pay out of your own pocket." Norman felt bad that he took advantage of the free food situation and ruined a good thing for everyone else.

After confronting both of the boys who were involved with the jaw-breaking incident, Norm felt smug and arrogant about the situations, but he had accomplished something that he had set out to do. If it wasn't for those two jokers who created a short snag in his life, he would have never become a bodybuilder and power weightlifter. The interest of harming either of those two children of God had finally disappeared.

Norman was one of 3,000 graduating students in the final class to ever walk the halls inside the Allentown High School under that name. In 1961 the high school's name was changed to William Allen.

CHAPTER 3
A RECRUIT ON THE PEDESTAL

Trench-digging was not what Norman pictured himself doing for the rest of his life. One morning he marched up the steep post office steps to visit with a recruiter. In those days they usually came looking for you. Norman had thought seriously about the Marine Corps, the branch that every tough guy wanted to join to impress the chicks. Unfortunately for him, the jarhead recruiters were on their coffee and doughnut break. The army recruiters signaled for him to stroll into their office to be vacuumed into a career of promises and guarantees. Norman just smiled and kept on walking. Machine guns, artillery, and battle zones weren't his idea of pleasure, and marching, jogging, and rifle drills were not his cup of tea either. Instead, he chose the United States Air Force, which he thought couldn't be all that bad. Little did he know that he picked the flyboys branch that was filled with marching and jogging, especially at the beginning.

Norman went home after signing his life away. Now he had the hardest job of all; telling his parents about the start of his day.

"You did what?" exclaimed his mother.

"I've passed the military test, and my high school diploma is in a safe place," answered Norman. "All I need to do is to pack my duffle bag. I leave tomorrow, Ma, and nobody's going to stop me." The recruits were going to be bussed to Philadelphia to be sworn in the following day, and then it was off to San Antonio for eight weeks of basic training.

Dorothy Irene screamed, "You should be going to college. I'm telling you you're never going to amount to nothing. Wait 'til your father hears about this."

"I'm over eighteen, and I already signed the papers, Ma," said Norman. "Let me live my own life."

When Henry arrived home from work, Dorothy started yapping at him, "Wait 'til you hear what your son did today. Go ahead and tell your father, Mr. Big Shot." Henry was very disappointed when he heard the news. He wanted his son to follow in his own footsteps and be a part of his trade. They were just waiting on an opening in the plumbers union.

Norman thought that it was going to be great getting away from home, just like most kids at that age. He left for San Antonio the next day. The blue duffle bag he was carrying had two changes of clothing, including an Emmaus Health Club sweatshirt that he wanted to wear once he reached Lackland Air Force Base. He also brought along his own survival kit: protein powder and dozens of vitamins. He didn't realize that they would confiscate everything.

The recruits were introduced to their drill instructor before they even got the chance to take their first breath of fresh Texas air. Sergeant Gidrey was approximately five feet tall in military-issued combat boots, but he had a voice that was ten times louder than any recruit standing in front of him. Right from the start the DI would shout military lingo (including many four-letter words) into the ears of the newly enlisted members at point blank range.

"I'm your mother, your father, your uncle, and your brother," screamed the DI. "You're here for the next eight weeks, and whatever I tell you to do, you will do! You will have no time in my force to do anything but wake up in the morning and go through my basic training drills and exercises. Then at nighttime you'll be too tired to do anything else. Once in a while you will get mail, so I do suggest that you all write back home to your mothers. And don't get any silly ideas of writing back to me because of what I said in my opening statement. That's already been done."

The next day Norman's drill instructor laughed when they shipped his bag of tricks back home and gave him the name Health Boy right off the bat.

The barracks of Sergeant Gidrey's platoon were shared by guys from all over the country. They were all there to stay for the next eight weeks with no escape routes—or at least that's what the recruits believed at the time.

During the first week the troops were trying to adapt to the ear-piercing sound of reveille and the act of moving around very rapidly even before dawn. The recruits had to put on their uniforms, make a tight rack so a quarter would bounce five inches in the air off the blanket, and be out on the street in platoon formation in a matter of minutes. One morning the DI started roll call, and one of the recruits' name was not heard after being called upon twice. So the screaming sergeant instructed the boys to start their morning procedure all over again, from in bed to out on the road for roll call in a designated time limit. It seemed like they repeated this military drill about fifty times. Breakfast was out of the question.

"You knuckleheads better find your missing colleague, or we'll be doing the same thing tomorrow bright and early!" exclaimed the drill instructor. Dumping toilet water on the missing recruit the next night in his rack cured him of any future tardiness.

Not all of the Air Force recruits could make the transformation from civilian life to listening to a strict, screaming DI giving out orders all day long. In fact, one of the guys in Norman's platoon just couldn't adapt to the military life, so he figured out how to purchase his ticket home. Just before a morning inspection, this recruit took a dump in his military-issued underwear and put them back into his duffle bag. Their bags had to be prepared properly with their gear and tied in the exact manner that the sergeant instructed for inspection. The DI came through and knocked over most of the duffle bags onto the racks. When the shorts fell out of that kid's bag, it was an undesirable sight, and the smell was putrid.

After the inspection was completely finished the sergeant yelled out, "I know what one certain person in my platoon is going to be wearing for our dinner date."

Besides all the marching and exercise drills on the physical training field, Norman still made time for his real body nourishment after lights-out. Between the double bunks he would do dips to build up his shoulder and chest muscles. Hand-clapper push-ups on the floor were another great exercise to get the blood flowing. He even persuaded the squad leaders to work out with him after the lights went out. But one night the sergeant came storming into the barracks and caught Norman in the act.

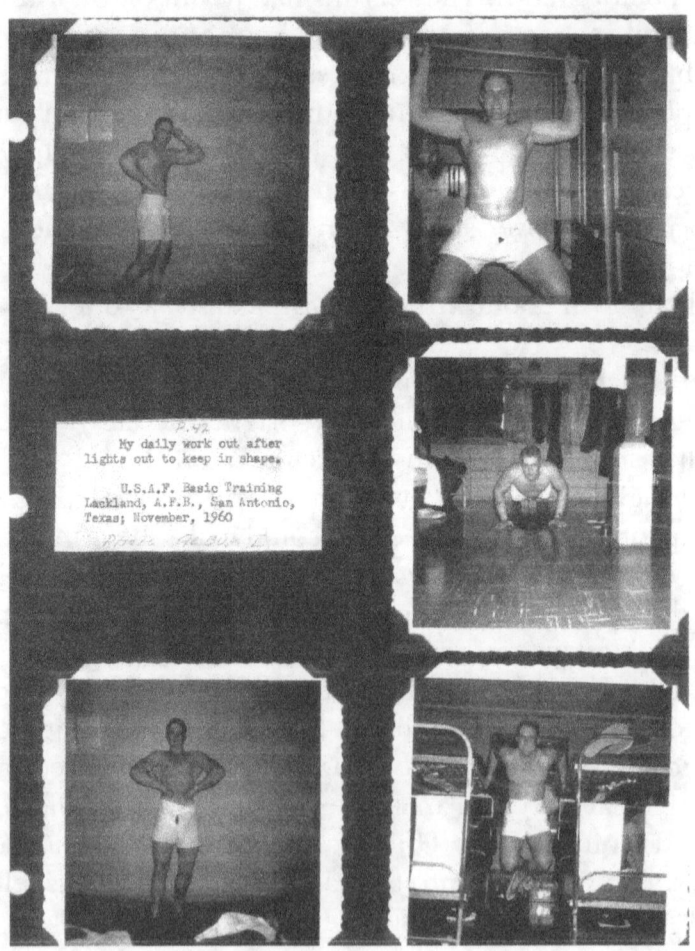

"Are you nuts, boy?" asked the drill instructor. "You should be sleeping. I guess you proved me wrong. Maybe we aren't wearing you out enough during the day."

About three weeks or so went by, and all the troops were out on the drill pad doing their daily routine exercises. The drill sergeant observed his recruits, knowing it would take some extra work to get them to perform like a precision-tuned, well-oiled machine. There would have to be a certain amount of tweaking done along the way. The troops still had numerous things to learn to get ready for the big show, and final inspection day wasn't that far off.

A cocky exercise instructor who the boys called Mr. Fit was on his front-view platform leading the training session that day.

"Mr. Rauch, fall out of ranks and step up to my platform on the double!" exclaimed the exercise instructor. "You were out of sync with the rest of the troops on the last two drills. I want uniformity amongst my squads. Give me five laps around the grinder in double-time fashion. Ready? Move out!" This guy rubbed all the recruits the wrong way, and he knew that Norman hated to run with a passion.

Norman didn't budge a step.

"Wait just one minute," yelled Norman's drill instructor, sticking up for him. "Why don't you challenge Health Boy to another task—something that I could put a small wager on?"

Norman Rauch yelled out, "I challenge you to push-ups. Whatever you can do, I'll pass it by fifty, or I'll run this track all day."

The exercise leader hastily took the challenge but was abruptly shut down by Health Boy. Norman did 105 push-ups to the exercise instructor's measly fifty-one. The DI got such a kick out of this that he ordered him to lead the exercises the following day on the platform. Health Boy made such a good impression that he was told to stay on his pedestal to train the troops for the rest of basic training. He was also chosen by his peers to be barracks chief.

Besides himself, there was only one other recruit who was missing from the drill and exercise line-up on the pad. The guy who had crapped his shorts was at last found on all fours, ramming his head into the barrack walls, acting like a sheep. It seemed that he was bucking for an inadaptable discharge.

After the eight weeks of basic training, Norman Rauch landed at Truax Field Air Defense Base in Madison, Wisconsin, for his first military assignment. The Air Force-enlisted personnel arrived in a much cooler climate than what they were used to. It was the end of December, and there were heavy piles of snow on the ground everywhere they looked. In the 327th Fighter Group barracks on base, Norman didn't see one familiar face, but he had no problem making friends. He knew that fellowshipping was part of his religious curriculum. A guy by the name of Leo was one of the first men Norman made an acquaintance with. He was also from Allentown, Pennsylvania, and had the nickname of Rocky.

"My last name is Rauch," stated Norman in his unforgettable bold voice. "Quite a few people pronounce it 'Rausch' with an S in the middle, but there is no S, and the CH on the end together makes the K sound. It's one of your basic peculiar English phonics rules. So in other words, my name sounds like Rauk or Rock."

"Well, you're built more like a rock than I am," gasped Leo. "I think that all the guys here on base should start calling you ROCKY. How about Big Rocky?" The name stuck, and Norman was very proud of it. From then on Leo was known as Little Rocky and Norman was Big Rocky.

Rocky continued to take his work-out sessions very seriously. In March of 1961, he entered the Wisconsin State Championship in Manitowoc. He not only won the event, but he also broke three state records. The two best heavyweight lifters in the state couldn't believe their eyes! They were dazed and confused. "Where did this guy come from anyway?" one of them asked. Rocky had been a complete unknown until then. He cleaned and jerked 360 pounds, pressed 270 pounds, and snatched 235 for a grand total of 865 pounds, breaking the three-lift records in his weight category. Everyone cheered and went crazy when superstar Big Rocky arrived back on base.

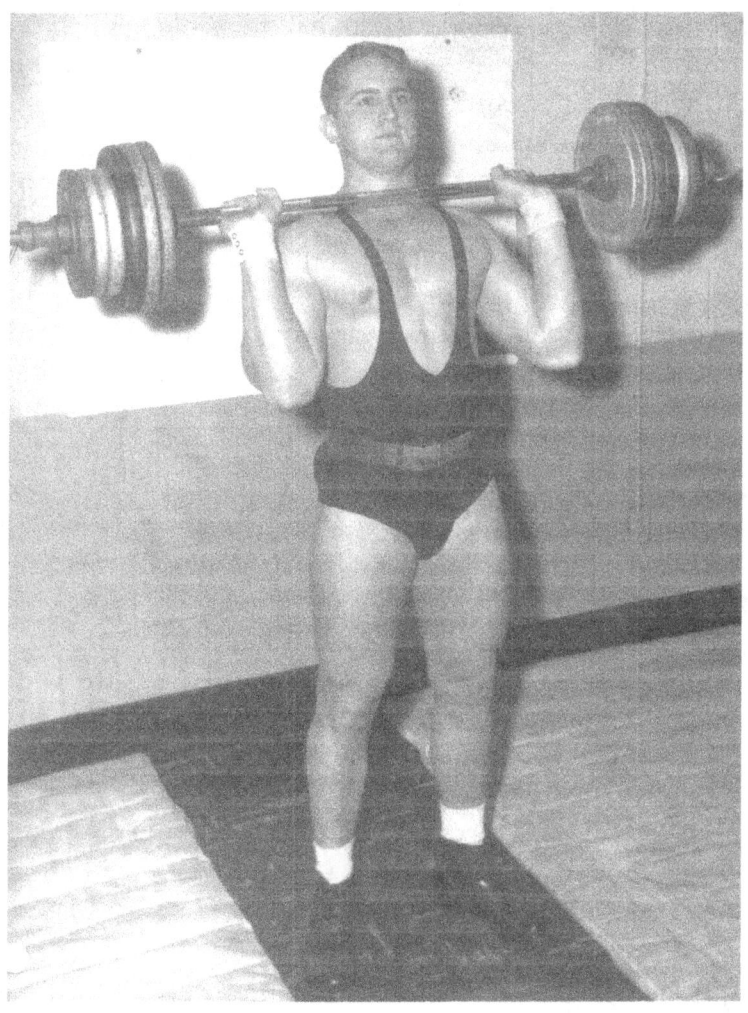

Rocky went on to win the Illinois/Iowa State Championship and everything he entered after that. The Air Force finally got wind of this and was very interested in his lifting ability. The first year on the base, he was given the duty of working in the service club. Putting on special activities such as dances and celebrations for the flyboys was part of his job.

Once he made a name and reputation for himself, his duties were made even easier. Rocky advanced to the position of towel boy, working in the base gymnasium. He not only handed out towels to trainees, but he also worked in the massage department on VIPs. After winning a number of weightlifting championships, he knew that he had it made in the Air Force.

Working out in the gym was another one of his duties. The good Lord was looking out for the boy when he passed by the Marine Corps Recruiting Office that day when nobody was home.

Basically, Rocky had three main jobs to do to fulfill his duty load each day. He had to work out hard to become the strongest airman that this military branch had ever seen. They wanted him to eat anything his heart desired anytime he wanted, as long as it was filled with protein. He was also given the task of handing out towels to whomever needed one. What a great gig!

One evening while working as a bouncer at a popular bar in Madison, Rocky met his first wife, Jade. When she accepted his strong masculine hand for a dance, she stood upright to the tune of five foot ten inches tall with a full-figured build, weighing approximately 185 pounds. Rocky started to tell Jade a little bit about his background. They exchanged glances and conversation throughout the night, even as Rocky continued to perform his work duties.

In June of 1962, Norman and Jade were pronounced man and wife until death split them apart (although in some situations cheating, lying, and lack of trust in each other could serve the same purpose).

Rocky had a weightlifting competition in Chicago and brought his new bride along for the ride. Director Bob Taffman walked up to him and said sarcastically in front of them both, "Why did you go and do a stupid thing like that? I hope you don't let this marriage get in the way of your weightlifting career."

If looks could kill, Taffman would have had piercing daggers shot into every part of his body. Jade's comeback was, "You'd better watch your step, mister, because I have coffee with some high-ranking government officials every morning. On second thought, I don't need them to back me up. Come on, buster. Let's dance!"

A year later the Air Force was watching every move that Mr. Rauch made. The Olympic Games were coming up in 1964. He won the Air Defense Command Championship in 1963, along with every other contest the Air Force had to offer. The last competition was the Air Force Finals in Wichita Falls, Texas, which he had no problem winning. After that, Rocky was treated like royalty.

The Air Force flew Rocky to Denver, Colorado, to use his skills to qualify for the Olympic tryouts, which would be held the following year in New York at the World's Fair. He won the prestigious match in Denver and was chosen to lift in the North American Championship in Minneapolis, Minnesota, with competitors from Mexico, Cuba, the United States, and Canada.

During his second snatch lift, Rocky hyperextended his elbow and severely tore his forearm muscle. He dropped the enormous barbell weight and knew immediately that something was drastically wrong. He shoved open the training room door with his good arm, and one of the competitors said, "It looks like I'm finally going to be able to beat you, Mr. Rauschie." After using the proper ointment and wrapping his arm in an Ace bandage, Rocky went back out in the limelight and power cleaned and jerked 300 pounds. That lift won him the heavyweight division championship.

The injured weightlifter was escorted to a nearby hospital immediately to have x-rays taken to determine the extent of the damage. There were no broken bones found, and his arm was put in a cast. Back on base, the military specialists cut the cast off and also took x-rays. Then they put another cast back on his forearm and sent him back down to San Antonio to go through extensive therapy. Rocky had already qualified to go to the World's Fair to try out for the Olympic team, but this forearm injury prevented him from doing so.

Rocky blamed God for holding him back. "Why do you put me in these situations that deny me the right to achieve the goals that not many of your other children would even have a shot at, Lord?" thought Rocky.

The specialists in Texas wanted to do exploratory surgery, but the airman would not sign the medical forms. Rocky tipped the scales at a grand total of 297 pounds, trying to reach another personal goal of 300. Since his blood pressure was high, his doctor put him on a strict diet to lose weight immediately. He walked into the hospital wearing a size 19½ shirt, size 46 trousers, and a size 56 coat. The next three months in the therapy hospital ward were going to be a long haul.

At first his diet consisted of 1,500 calories per meal three times a day. Then it was reduced to 1,000 calories and finally to 750. For a body of that mass, 1,500 calories per meal was like a prisoner restricted to consuming only bread and water. Rocky's hearty appetite sometimes required three steaks and a half-loaf of bread at one sitting. Another meal might have been limited to a dozen ears of corn and a quart of milk to wash the kernels down. He was averaging two gallons of milk per day. With any meal, a half-gallon of ice cream was necessary for dessert to complete his forced eating habits. For the first month or so, Rocky's health was in danger because of his high blood pressure and his young age. The hospital nurses measured and weighed everything that he ate.

After being discharged, Rocky walked out of the hospital with a sense of pride. He felt like a brand new vehicle off of the assembly line—like a VW beetle, not a step van. The young man felt much better, and his reflexes were a lot quicker at the astonishing weight of 192 pounds. He had lost 105 pounds in three months. In a strength and health magazine, an article was printed called "The Amazing Story of Norman Rauch" by the one and only Bob Taffman. It explained his unique physical structure and displayed before and after photographs.

The last stretch of the ride home to Madison was in a Greyhound Bus. Rocky telephoned his wife Jade to meet him at the bus terminal. While waiting for his ride home, he thought about the new clothes he had to buy. His shirt size had shrunk to a 16½, his trousers were a size 32, and his new coat size was 44. The pretty girls all took notice of this handsome man still in his Air Force uniform.

Rocky just stood with great posture and a partial smirk on his face while Jade walked past him and in and out of the bus station twice. Then she walked up to Rocky and asked, "Excuse me, sir. Did you happen to see any other Air Force personnel step off of that last bus?"

Trying to keep a straight face and altering his husky voice slightly, Norman Rauch spoke, "Are you looking for your husband, madam?"

Jade's eyeballs almost popped out of their sockets when her scrawny husband spoke. "Why didn't you tell me that you lost so much weight?" She could feel other women giving her husband the eye as they spoke. "Why did you keep this a big secret?"

"I don't know," stated Norman. "I guess I just wanted to see that surprised look on your face when I arrived home."

Already a little jealous, Jade said, "I don't know if I like you being thin. You will get too much attention from the opposite sex."

Norman was already thinking about new goals to set for himself. He felt stronger and more flexible weighing just two-thirds of what he weighed not that long ago. In the 198-pound category Rocky could out-lift himself from when he weighed 297. Everyone thought that was phenomenal.

After being out of the service for some time, the weightlifting organization had come out with a 242-pound weight class (heavyweight).

In 1968 Rocky was training in the 242-pound category, entering every possible competition that he could. This was the era that anabolic steroids came into the realm on a national level. In Chicago, Illinois, Rocky cleaned and jerked 400 pounds, giving him a grand total of 1,000 pounds for all three scheduled lifts. He was the very first lifter from the state of Wisconsin to achieve that unbelievable total for the press, snatch, and clean and jerk weight lifts.

In around 1970 Norman Rauch went on to the Junior National Championships in Long Island, New York. He needed to clean and jerk 405 pounds to beat one of his highly-ranked competitors and win the competition. After putting up a bit of a struggle, Rocky jerked the weight over his head and won the match! Winning this tournament played a significant role in the heavyweight's career.

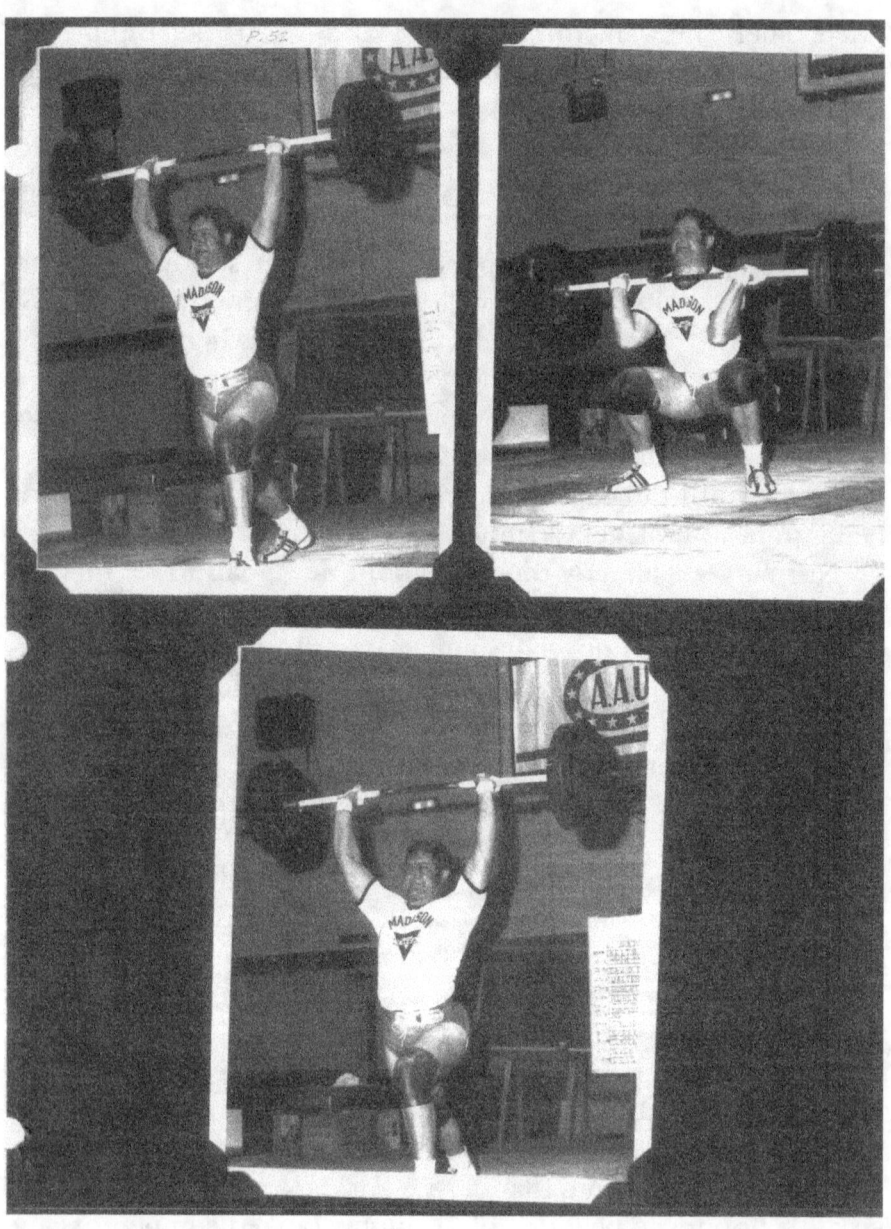

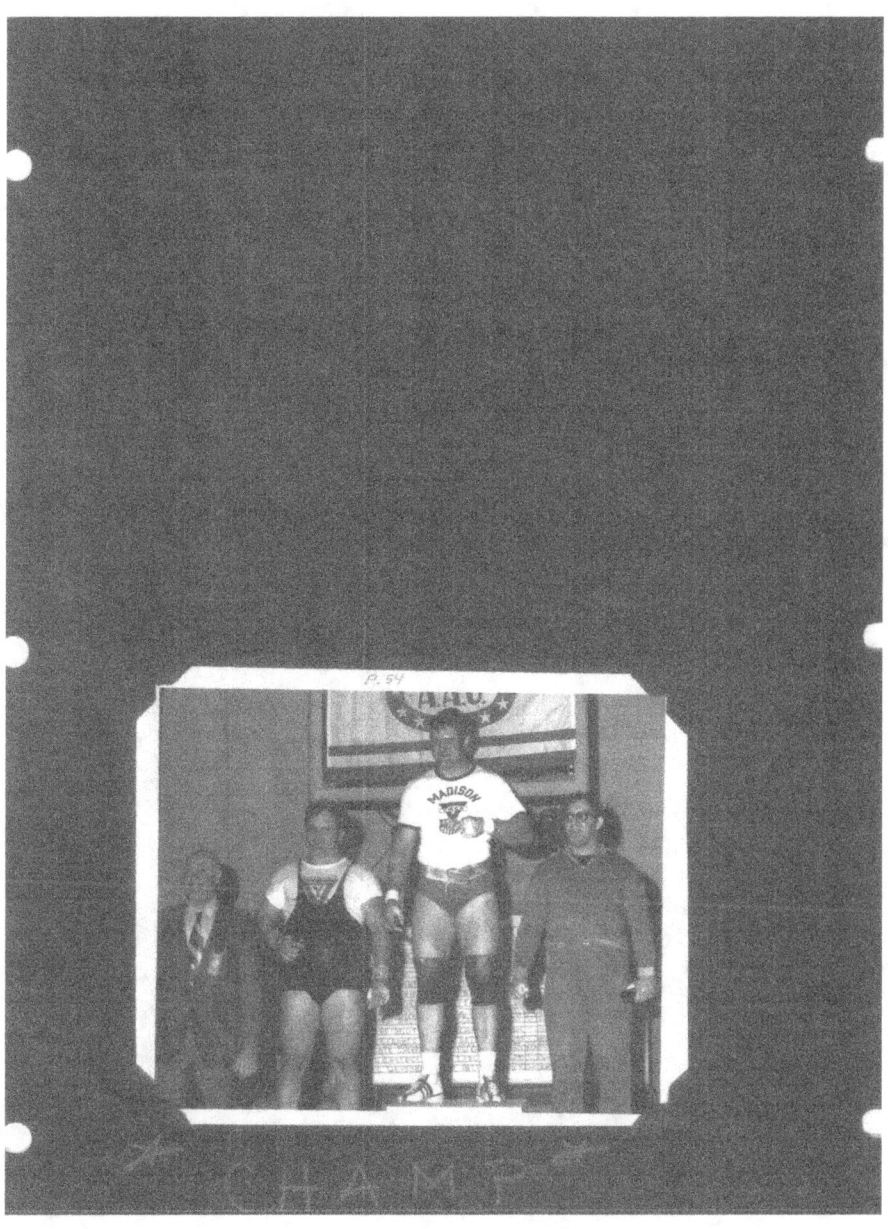

CHAPTER 4
STEWS, 'ROIDS, AND STRIPPERS
(PARTY TIME)

Winning the Junior National Championship was one of the highlights of Norman Rauch's weightlifting career. This event launched his professional pursuit even farther by giving the young man the opportunity to enter the Senior Nationals. In 1970 this weightlifting exhibition was ranked the NUMBER 1 top Olympic lifting contest in the United States.

Arriving in Culver City, California, for the professional competition, Rocky checked into the Hacienda Hotel. This was a highly-rated housing center for the Senior National heavyweights. The widely advertised event was to take place at the convention center in Culver City. That afternoon the athletes were able to take a short tour of the "behind the scenes" warm-up area where the nationally-televised tournament was to be held in less than twenty-four hours.

At qualification time, the weightlifters would warm up their muscles and get comfortable with their movements before taking the three starting lifts. The Olympic lifters would then be granted three attempts for each of the three categories. At the time, Robert Bernarski was the premier lifter in the heavyweight class, pressing 400 pounds, cleaning and jerking 480 pounds, and snatching 360. The heavyweight and super heavyweight matches were the highlight of the competition. That's when the convention center would be packed to its fullest capacity. Everyone wanted to see the big guys lift.

Meanwhile, back at the Hacienda Hotel, a group of TWA airline stewardesses were shuffling around up on the top floor. The gorgeous dolls were waiting on their orders to be placed somewhere in the friendly skies so that they could start shaking their tails for the passengers. Rocky and the muscle-bound pack of wolves just happened to create a marvelous brainstorm when they returned back to their rooms.

"Hey guys, what do you say we strip down to our bare asses, drape these bed sheets around our bodies," suggested one of the crew members, "and pay those stews a close visit? Maybe we'll even get some tail!" The flashing adventure was about to unfold.

The entire pack started traipsing through the halls and up to the highest level, according to the elevator clockwise dial. They looked as if they were going to a toga party.

After arriving on the top floor of the Hacienda, the elevator door opened, and Rocky was shoved outside into the hall without his bed sheet. The rest of the bunch had kept their clothes on underneath their sheets. Rocky was in his birthday suit in an unfamiliar hallway with nothing in sight but an ashtray on a stand with sand in it for camouflage. The only thing that he could think of at the moment was to dump the sand and cigarette butts out of the metal tray to try to cover himself up.

A couple of stewardesses came around a corner, put their hands to their mouths, chuckled and snickered a bit, and continued down the carpet path to their destination. At the same time Rocky was pushing every button in sight to get back in the elevator car. The one that he'd been pushed out of was in the "stuck" mode, but he heard a little jingle and saw a green light come on. Then the elevator door opened, and he got inside.

Instead of it stopping at his floor, the steel boxcar continued to go all the way down to the first floor lobby. He could hear the little jingle from inside the car this time. The sliding door opened to maybe a hundred hotel patrons in view from the cathedral ceiling main hotel lobby. Rocky was standing there with nothing to do but salute the crowd while holding the ashtray in front of himself, his shiny buttocks reflecting off the full-length mirror behind him. This scene eventually became the talk of the entire competition.

The senior weightlifters took their profession seriously. They knew when they could screw around and when they had to get down to business. When it came time to weigh in, the muscular lifters had to pay the consequences if they were even half a pound over their weight limit. You could either try to do a lot of spitting or take a steam shower. Running was out of the question because it would take too much strength and endurance from their massive bodies. Every bodybuilding weightlifter had two chances to weigh in.

Rocky failed his first weigh-in attempt a few hours before the warm-up event was to take place. He needed to lose a pound and a half. Somehow, he made the weight cut by weighing in the second time at 241 pounds 11 ounces.

There were more Olympic lifters in the 242-pound weight class than in any of the other divisions. At one time not so very long ago, muscular weightlifters were averaging around 1,000 pounds for their three best attempts out of the three different categories. Now with more knowledge of tendon strength instead of muscle size, the Olympic lifters were pumping over 1,100 pounds of solid iron.

It was time for the warm-up procedures to begin, and the cameras were starting to roll at the convention center. The requirements were for a back brace and a singlet bodysuit to be worn. Some of the lifters wore instep strap shoes with elevated heals for the squat or split-style snatch lift.

Rocky opened up with a 325-pound press and instantly jumped to 345 for the second lift. He missed the third warm-up attempt at the weight of 365 pounds. Some days the barbell would feel like a ton of bricks and other times like a feather in a cowgirl's sombrero. That's when you could break records!

Rocky was in the best shape of his life, and the weights felt good. He rubbed some chalk on his hands and cleaned the weight from the floor. Then, throwing his left leg behind his rear end, he got underneath the bar and lunged it upward to make the split-style snatch lift.

Rocky finished up his warm-up drills by doing a series of isometric and isotonic exercises. For isometrics, he pushed against a permanent object with all his might for ten seconds. He did ten repetitions before moving on to the isotonic lifts. He then did a series of lifting a bar from a lower pin to an upper pin on a weight rack and holding it there for fifteen seconds at a time. For these lifts, he needed to be very strong in the lower back and waist area, just like a young tree must have a thick trunk to be able to withstand the strong centrifugal force of a howling wind.

At the heart of the competition, Rocky accumulated a fantastic score. His superb finale press was 355 pounds, the split-style snatch was recorded at 305 pounds, and the clean and jerk was his best-ever score at 405.

Up until 1968, Rocky pursued his bodybuilding and weightlifting career the old-fashioned, natural way. He earned it by working hard and paying his dues. However, there was a rumor going around that if you wanted to go even further as a power lifter, you might want to inquire about a substance called the BIG D. Wanting to be in with the in-crowd, Rocky made an appointment with his local doctor to take a physical and was prescribed Dianabol on the spot with no questions asked. Even the specialists had no real statistics on the side effects of steroids.

No weightlifter wanted to fall behind the times, so just about everyone became attached to the "orals." Rocky swallowed two small blue tablets a day for an eight-week cycle. Then his instructions were to hold off for four weeks. Nobody was dropping dead or getting liver disease from the 'roids at the time, so Rocky and his peers thought they were being put to good use.

One would feel the surge from a prescribed group of fat-soluble organic compounds (steroids) in approximately three to four days. This would in turn increase your bodyweight, muscle size, and no-longer-natural strength. During the four-week off-cycle, the steroid user's strength would taper off, and the lifts would drop in weight. The weightlifter would hardly be able to wait to get back on them, especially if a match was coming up soon. He would try to gear the competitions toward the up-cycle, when the Olympic lifter would be at his peak.

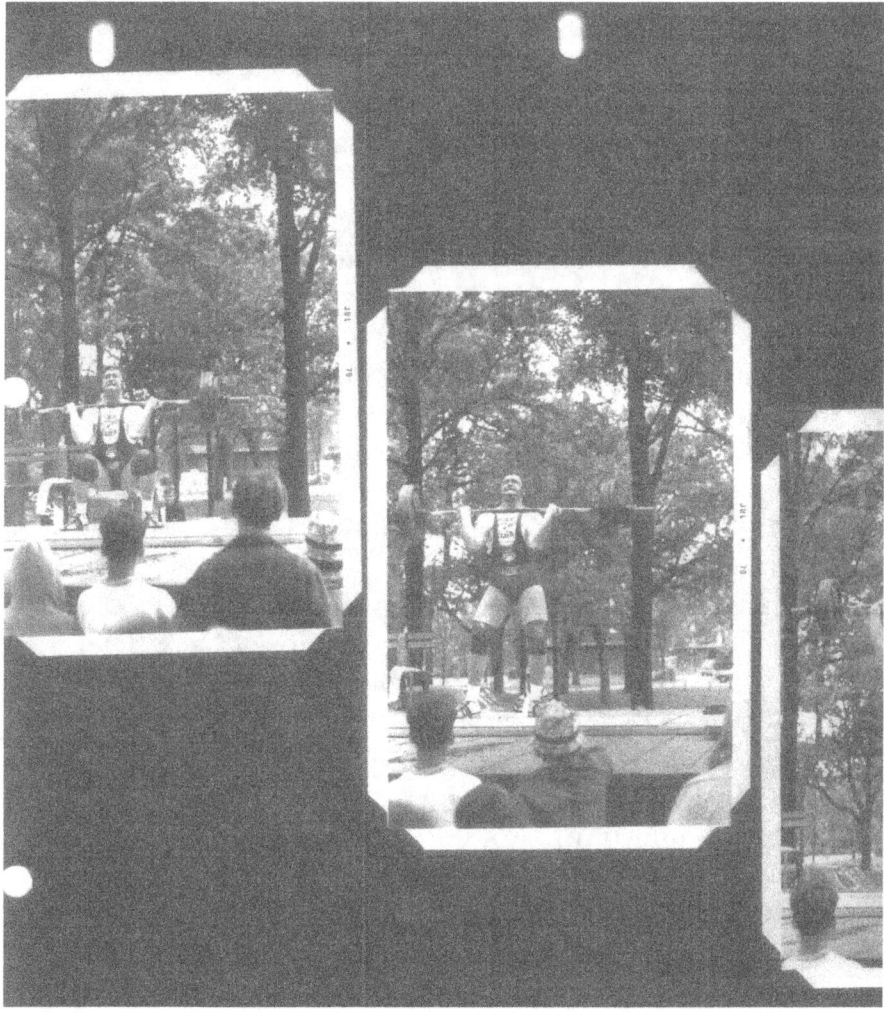

The steroid was invented by a German scientist during the Hitler regime. The commanding officers wanted to make their soldiers more aggressive. At the same time, when soldiers were wounded, they would be transported to a hospital, and their fragment lacerations would repair themselves much faster. Later, when soldiers were released from concentration camps with malnutrition, steroids were used to speed up the body functions to a normal level.

What the specialists didn't know about the drugs back then or in the early 1970s was that they could cause toxic build-up on the liver with extended use, and they could speed up your metabolism, which would increase muscle tissue at a faster rate. Dianabol was a muscle– and strength-enhancer that in time would suppress the immune system and could have an effect on the pancreas.

There were many local practitioners were associated with weightlifters who would hand out oral steroids sometimes, for the right price. It was like a kid opening his bag wide for candy after doing a trick at Halloween time. But still nobody would go around and advertise this fairly new secret. It was all kept very hush-hush for some time. Rocky finally understood where his father was coming from when he made the statement about cheating on your body. "You will pay the consequences in the long run." Maybe his dad was right. Rocky knew deep down that his father would not be very proud of him if he ever found out.

One morning Rocky woke up and noticed two medium-sized boils, one on his shoulder and one on his lower back. They were lanced by the local doctor, but no blood work was done. A few weeks later Rocky spotted another boil near his nostril. A short time after that his eye became swollen and the entire side of his face puffed up like a small balloon. He was put on antibiotics and treated for an infection. Two more huge boils popped up on his stomach and one on the back of the leg. Finally, the local practitioner said that this situation was very abnormal and sent Rocky to visit an internist in Madison, Wisconsin. Jade was very worried and went along to get some answers.

After a series of blood tests were taken, the specialist entered the waiting area and said, "Mr. Rauch, I hate to alarm you, but the results of this blood study do not look good. You have a severely deteriorated liver similar to that of an acute alcoholic. Do you drink excessively?"

"Just an occasional beer with the guys," answered Rocky.

"Your white blood count is also very low," explained the doctor. "What have you been doing?"

"Well, I do take a couple of small blue pills a day to enhance my weightlifting career," admitted Rocky, feeling down and a bit guilty.

"What are these pills called?" asked the specialist. "Do they have a name?"

"Dianabol," stated Rocky. The doctor immediately looked this medicine up in his most recent medical journal.

"You are consuming a drug that is referred to as an anabolic steroid, Mr. Rauch," he said. "The possible side effects include cardiovascular problems, high blood pressure, liver damage, liver cancer, suppressed immune system, and increased metabolism. Should I go on?" Rocky just shook his head in disbelief. "Definitely do not drink alcoholic beverages of any kind, and lay off of the blue pills, Mr. Rauch, or you will drop dead. Do I make myself clear? Eat well-balanced meals, and I will see you again in exactly thirty days."

Workouts were getting harder and harder because of the painful boils. When the thirty-day period was over, Rocky went back to the specialist to see if anything had improved. The doctor came back with the test results and said that the liver was perfectly normal, the immune system was fine, and there was no staph infection. It was like magic, as if nothing had ever happened to begin with. The specialist stated that the liver is one of the few organs in your body that can repair itself and that Rocky was very fortunate that they had caught the problem in time.

Rocky consented to do an experiment with the doctor. He was to consume only one five-milligram blue pill a day for thirty days, and they would see what the outcome would be at the next visit.

Another thirty days went by, and he went back to the clinic once again for blood tests. The liver showed signs of deterioration, and the white blood count was way down, but there was no staph infection. "Well, I believe we have the problem narrowed down, Mr. Rauch," explained the specialist. "You should quit taking the steroids. Once your liver is completely destroyed, you're as good as gone. It's as simple as that. With your white count down, your immune system is weakened, and the body is going to be susceptible to any kind of an infection. Who knows what might happen?"

"Well, if I have to quit taking the fuel for my internal fire, I won't be able to compete anymore," answered the broken-down Rocky. "All the super giants are on STEROIDS."

"I can't tell you what to do, Mr. Rauch," stated the doctor. "It's your choice. If I were your personal therapist, I might say to continue with the drug and be every weightlifting fan's hero for maybe another six months, or you could possibly do something else with your life, such as teaching younger kids the sport the natural way. But I'm not your psychiatrist. The decision is yours for the making."

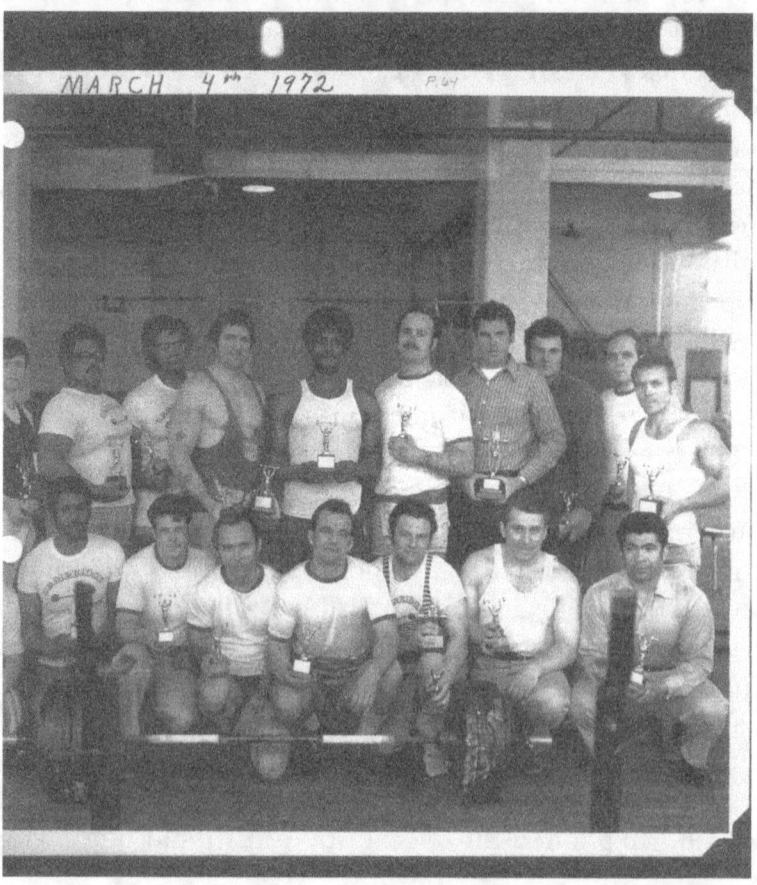

It wasn't worth the hassle of dealing with the boils, and certainly the thought of dropping out of commission was out of the question. So Rocky made his decision immediately to stop using steroids. His weight dropped from 250 to 220 pounds practically overnight. He continued to lift weights and became runner-up in the Junior Mr. Wisconsin Championship for both 1971 and 1972. He decided to bodybuild again (not power weightlifting) without the use of help from his little blue friends.

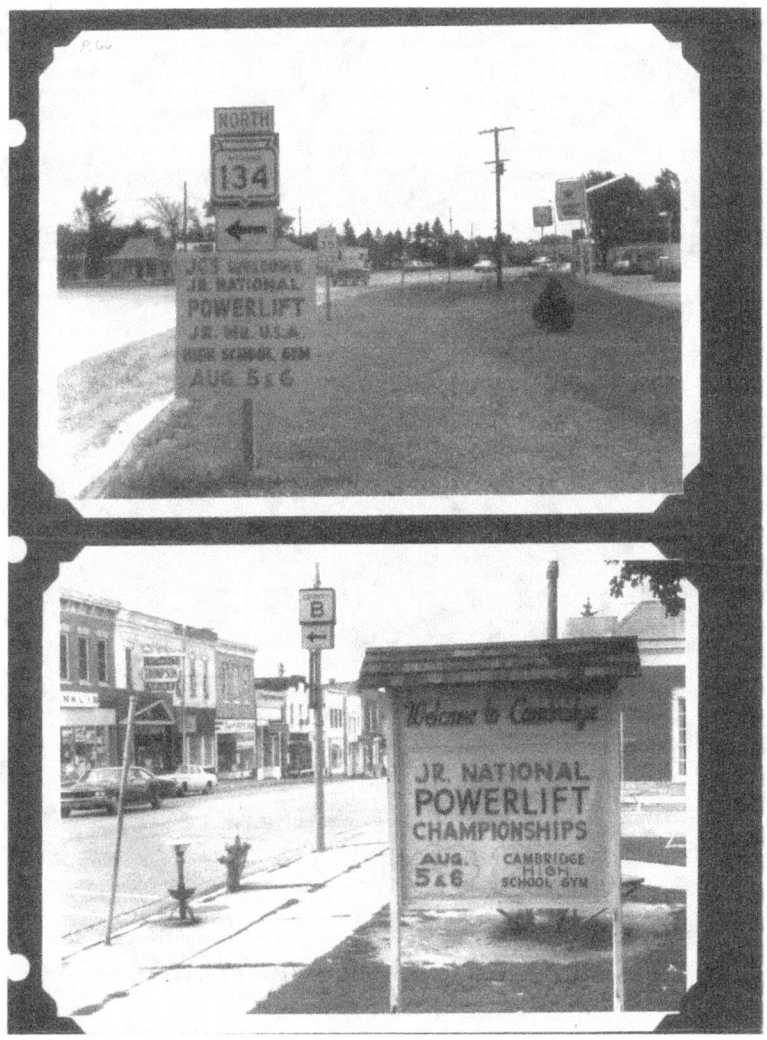

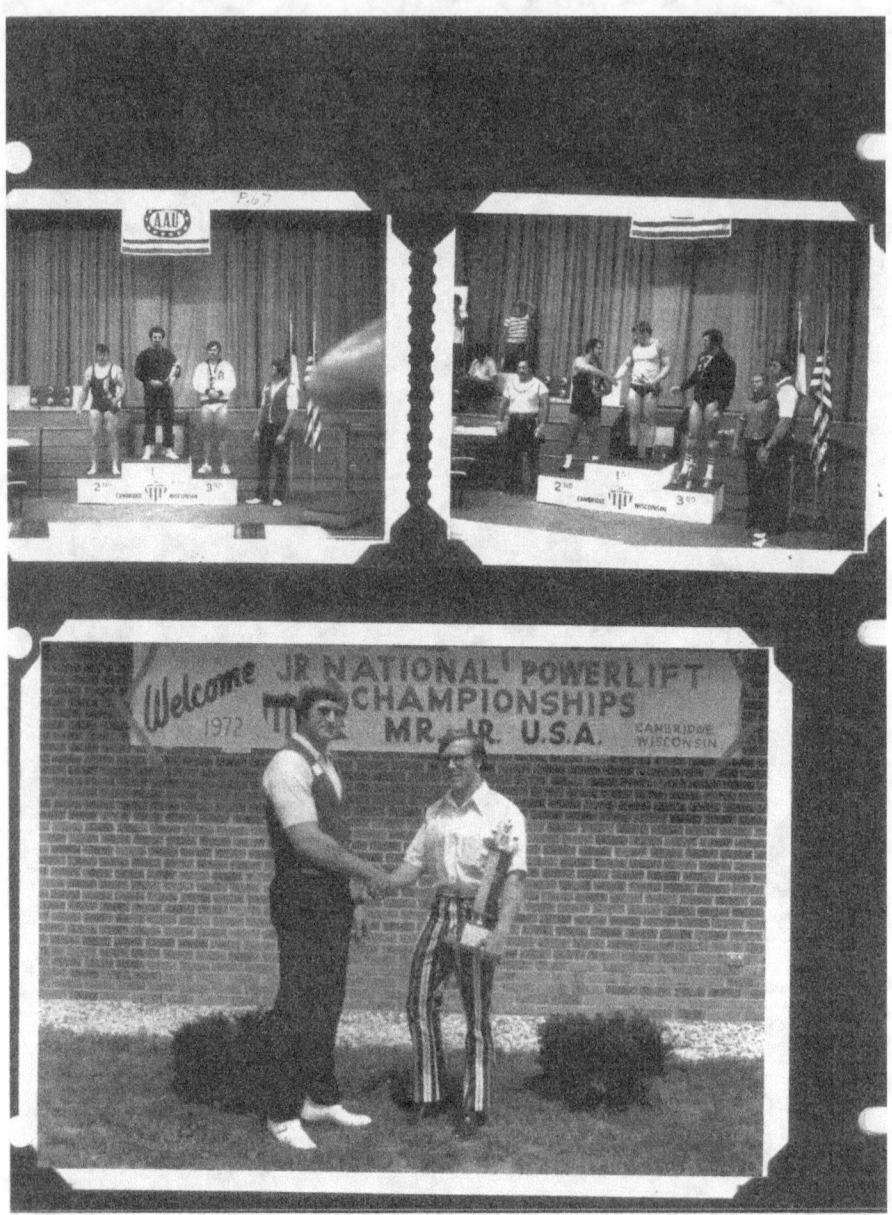

Rocky always pondered if he was on this earth because someone believed in him. He thought that the good Lord knew what
he had in mind for Rocky before he was even born, so his number

wasn't up yet! Rocky gave up the sport of bodybuilding a while after he met a gal by the name of Kerry Fitzpatrik. She just idolized him, and they hit it off very well together. At the time, Rocky was still in a marriage that was on very shaky ground. He spent most of his time in the gym when he was still working out, and Jade was always dedicated to her job.

Kerry worked in the Madison school district with the slower-learning children. At first Norman and Kerry spent some time together in the afternoons, and gradually the relationship got heavier. Jade soon realized that her husband was cheating on her and filed for a divorce. She told him that he had exactly two weeks to get all of his stuff out of her house.

Rocky had to make a living just like everyone else, so he worked for the Benson Pump Company out of Rockford, Illinois. His occupation was a wholesale distributor salesman who had to do some traveling throughout the Southern Wisconsin area. He had the gift of gab while talking to his customers, both on the telephone and in person. His company manufactured whirlpool tubs, well pump equipment, swimming pool materials and supplies, and much more. One day as he was driving back to the Benson home office, Rocky just couldn't keep his mind off of the past, being married to Jade with a daughter, and being stationed in Biloxi, Mississippi in the Air Force. He had plenty of time to let his mind wander back into the 1960s.

I remember it well, living by the lake in Cambridge, Wisconsin, with my wife Jade and a daughter soon to come. We owned a screened-in garage that was a workout center for me and all of my buddies. The estate was only 100 feet from Lake Ripley, where we could run and go skinny-dipping after our workouts. It was a very nice, quiet area of around 600 people all having lake rights. I still remember catching some huge large-mouths off of our huge pier.

I re-enlisted back into the United States Air Force in Mississippi and was in the Grounds Repair Unit. It was 1965, and my wife Jade was pregnant with my first child. The Vietnam era was presented along with American muscle cars and itsy-bitsy, teeny-weeny yellow polka dot bikinis.

I recall when I was exactly ten years of age, out of nowhere a tiny baby boy popped out of my mother's oven and eventually gained all of the attention in the household. But the week that Charlie took his first breath in God's creation, I was so astonished that I ran to school and told my fourth grade teacher Mrs. Bomb the good news. She was invited over to see baby Charlie that evening. Three weeks later all the aunts and cousins came to pamper Charlie, and I was pushed off to the sidelines.

I could not take any more of the excitement, so a red farmer's handkerchief was yanked out of my father's dresser drawer. All my belongings were gathered up, and I attached the full knotted-up hanky to my bamboo fishing pole. Then I was off like a rocket ship at the base of Cape Canaveral. All alone I flew down Lumber Street past Aunt Kate and Uncle Willie's house, not having a clue to where I was going. Some days you just don't feel like sticking around to see someone else get all of the attention.

It just happened to be around 3:30 p.m., and my stomach was starting to growl. I knew that supper was always on time at 5:00 p.m. sharp. So I decided to take a short break from running away and to go back home to feed my gut. I still remember the look on my mother's face when I got back, apologized, and asked what was for supper. She was about ready to bend my bamboo pole into the shape of a question mark over my head as she said, "Your favorite meal, son: a spinach and broccoli casserole." After that day I decided to put up with that little shit of a brother named Charlie. But I still went on to tease and torment the little guy with a Frankenstein mask that I found in the basement's treasure of junk.

Things weren't going so well after I was in the Air Force again down in Biloxi. We still had many unpaid bills to straighten out in Wisconsin. I remember not being able to get any financial support. Jade's parents thought that I was an unstable bum moving from job to job a lot and then going back into the military. The service didn't pay much. We lived on cheap food like oatmeal and crackers for weeks. I felt that I had made another wrong decision. But you can't just walk away from the military life unless you go AWOL.

Jade and I discussed this matter over a drink one night and together we remembered that she still had a little bit of pull. She knew one of the state senators from when she was a secretary for the State of Wisconsin. Jade made a telephone call that pulled a series of strings, and I was released on a hardship discharge just like that. All I had to do was to verify that I had a full-time job waiting for me back home.

I can remember the exact words that my commanding officer said to me as I walked into the headquarters building to sign the discharge papers: "I hope that you never want to come back into the military."

My response was something like, "Why not?" even though I knew that this time it was going to be strictly civilian life for me from now on. The commander said, "Because you have 'PI' stamped on your records. That stands for 'political influence,' which means somebody through politics helped you to get out. Me and my fellow officers don't like that so much."

We left the base that day and eventually found an apartment in Madison, Wisconsin. We had already made the mistake of selling the house in Cambridge, so we couldn't go back there. I worked a few different low-paying jobs but was never very happy. So I called my father back in Pennsylvania and asked if there was anything he could do to help me out. Pops said that he could get me into the plumbers union making $10 to $12 an hour starting out. They would take around $5 a week out of my paycheck for union dues. That was big money back then.

So back around 1966 I went east to Pennsylvania to get established in the union and to live with my folks for a while. I called for my wife and daughter, who was three or four months old at the time, to come out there some time later. Just seeing my old buddies and working out at the YMCA in Pennsylvania again was just the ultimate kick out of life. I hung out with Bobby Bartholomew, who went on to place in the Olympics in 1968.

After being there for about six months I remember realizing that my marriage was going down the tubes. Now at this very moment I understand why. I was spending all of my time in the gym or going out with the boys. I won the Pennsylvania State Championship that year in the 198-pound weight category. My friend Bobby was competing on the World Championship team. I went to see him lift in York, Pennsylvania. Jade was going to hop on an airplane with the baby that next morning to visit her family back near Madison. I wasn't scheduled to be back until later on in the day. So I watched Bobby compete early and didn't feel like sticking around for the rest of the competition.

The hands on the kitchen clock struck 2:00 a.m. at home when I entered the room. I remember noticing two empty glasses on the kitchen table. The bedroom sounded inviting at the time, and I didn't think much about the glasses. Jade was in the other room, asleep.

The next thing I knew, the telephone was ringing, and I jumped out of bed half-asleep to answer it. To my surprise it was a stripper friend that Jade and I knew fairly well from one of the local clubs. She must have noticed me getting in late and wanted to tell me that my wife was playing kissy-face with Tom from the restaurant that they both worked at.

The stripper asked me if I was going to do anything about it. I told her that I was upset and just wanted to go for a walk to blow off some steam. She just lived right down the street and invited me over for coffee. A short time after I arrived at her place, the hot stripper asked me what I wanted: "Coffee, tea, or me?" I decided to choose the latter.

The next morning I overslept until about 7:40, knowing that Jade and my child would be boarding the plane at 8:00. I did the bunny hop out of the stripper's bed, grabbed my pants, and was off to the races. I remember breaking all speed limits trying to get to the airport. The airplane was just about ready for departure, but I was given permission to quickly say good-bye to my wife and kid.

Jade knew that I had spent the night with the stripper because the phone had woken her up, and she overheard the conversation. We argued for a couple of minutes about that and her being with Tom the previous night. I picked up my daughter, gave her a smooch on the cheek, and started to walk off the plane. Jade yelled at me that she and my kid were never coming back. Shaky and upset, I drove back to my parents' home and explained the entire situation to my mother and father. My mother just grinned and spoke, "I never did know that woman from the beginning. Stay here in Pennsylvania with us and live in your apartment. Don't go chasing after her. Hopefully she'll never come back."

Rocky put his mind at ease for the next couple of minutes while staring out of the driver's seat window, noticing that the scenery was starting to look a bit more familiar. For the rest of the drive back he just couldn't focus his thoughts on the present and what the future would bring. Norman still had this guilty feeling trapped inside of him.

I remember saying to my mother that Jade still had my daughter Sally Ann and I couldn't believe that she ran off like that. It was probably all my fault. Approximately six more months at the apartment was about all I could handle. Ma was paying all of my bills and banking all of my money. Depression started to set in, and I was feeling sorry for myself a lot. My drinking became heavier, and I quit lifting weights. I did run quite a bit to vent off steam when I was upset, even though I really hated running.

At the YMCA I joined the 100 Mile Club and ran so many 440-yard laps a day until I reached 100 miles. It took a couple of months to complete the task and to receive my grand award. It was a t-shirt that had "100 Mile Club" printed on the front. I guess my real goal at the time was to get down into the 181-pound weight category to start lifting again as a featherweight. I never did reach my goal. Around 185 pounds was as low as I could drop in weight.

Jade called one day and asked if I could hire the Allied Van Company to move all of her antiques and stuff back to Cambridge. Like a fool (as my mother called me), I did what my wife requested. A good friend by the name of Jeff Mayer helped me with the move but also accused me of being half-crazy. He said that I had it made where I was at and that I should not have been thinking about helping Jade out.

Well, eventually I did go back to Cambridge because I missed Sally Ann very much. I gave Jade a call when I arrived, and she said, "If you even think that we're going to get back together, you might just be in for a bit of a shock." Jade thought that I was crazy also and at first didn't want anything to do with me, until she found out from a lawyer that she could get a ton of money out of me because I made my residence in the same state. The courts slapped me with full child support papers.

After a while Jade granted me the pleasure of babysitting my child when she went off to work at her waitress job. I remember very clearly reading letters that I found in her dresser drawer from Tom the cook. They'd had an affair for two weeks here in Cambridge, Wisconsin!

I let that slide and started to become more successful by the day working for the Baker Manufacturing Company. I had my own company car, and Jade realized that I was doing pretty well for myself. We decided to get back together again as a family, which maybe worked out for about eight months. I continued to do what I did best at the time. Lifting weights again with my buddies and being a party animal came natural to me.

Another woman caught my eye along the way, and we were attracted to each other like magnets. Opposites attract. I wanted a romance and she didn't. She was happy with just the dating scene.

One day this girl called my home phone number, and Jade just happened to answer the telephone. Both women wanted to know who the other one was. Jade thought very quickly and said, "I am Norman's sister." I didn't tell this girl that I was married.

Well, this girl spilled her guts to my wife about our wonderful affair. Jade instantly wanted a divorce but found out not too long after that she was pregnant with my second child. Her doctor persuaded her to stay with me mainly for the children's sake. He was probably afraid that I might run back to Pennsylvania with no intention of paying child support. I was out to dinner with one of my dealers when Jennifer was born.

Jade and I eventually legally separated from each other in 1971.

When Norman arrived back in town, he nonchalantly drove past his home office building and parked on the street a few miles away. He walked up a flight of stairs and then down the bright red shag carpet runway along the side view of 250 antique pews. Before Norman reached the east side of the altar where there were numerous candles flickering, he genuflected while looking upward and made the sign of the cross. He then lit an unburned wick, got down on both knees, and stared at the colored candles. Norman looked up at the cathedral ceiling and poured his heart out. "Please forgive me, my Lord and Almighty Creator. I have sinned against you many times. Now I have nothing to show for what I have done. My family is gone, and I only have you left to turn to. I need your absolute forgiveness and your word that I won't burn in Hell!"

A man of the cloth put his right hand on Norman shoulder and said in a whisper, "I know who you are, my son. Have a little more patience with the Father in Heaven. Rome wasn't built in one day. Everything takes time."

CHAPTER 5
THE SECRET OF MANIPULATING
THE CUSTOMER

Phil Barrot was just finishing up with a bachelor's degree that he had earned from the University of Wisconsin-Madison. But Phil wanted more out of life. If you looked closely enough into his shiny green eyes, you could almost see the dollar-signs where his pupils should be. Phil thought that the best thing at the time would be to open a chain of massage parlors in the Madison area. He was going through the process of a divorce at the time, and he asked Rocky to move in with him to share some of the initial expenses.

The first thing that Phil did after settling down was to open his first massage parlor called the Rising Sun. In a small room at Phil's place, Rocky had his trophy case, an open closet for his clothes, and a military-type cot for sleeping on. That's all he really needed at the time, so all of his other possessions were stored. Rocky figured that this arrangement was temporary anyway because of the disgusting habits that Phil had inherited somewhere along the way. He would leave dirty dishes in the sink until mold formed, slurp cold spaghetti for breakfast, and leave the fans on all night because the sound helped him get to sleep. The two of them were like Felix and Oscar from *The Odd Couple*. Sometimes they didn't get along too well because Phil was basically a slob.

Rocky was still dating Kerry Fitzpatrik on and off. All he had to do was to say the word, and he could have moved into an elegant apartment with her. Kerry was loaded with money and even offered to pay for Rocky's education if he chose to take advantage of it. He just didn't want to get too attached to one woman.

One day, Rocky and Phil decided to hook up with a couple of women on the spur of the moment to go to a Cambridge Football game. Rocky escorted a blonde bombshell by the name of Ruby. She was a real knockout with the mental capacity of a chimpanzee. Phil brought an attractive dish who hung all over him and had no clue to how the game of football was played. During halftime Rocky's ex-wife Jade walked up to him and his date and asked them to leave. "You know your daughters are around here somewhere, and you shouldn't be seen with this blonde tootsie."

"I have every right in the world to be here," yelled Rocky. "I'm here with my friends because I love football. You have no business running my personal life."

A few minutes later, two-year-old Jennifer came into view and said, "Daddy, why don't you bring your blonde girlfriend over to my house, and we can all be a family?"

"I'm sure that would go over very well with your mother," snickered her dad.

Phil was starting to hire girls for his first massage parlor, the Rising Sun. Sexual manipulation was allowed by law, but penetration was prohibited. The proprietor would be shut down by the cops if the masseuse girls were caught in the act. The Rising Sun was more of a sexual massage parlor than a sports rub-down place. Sometimes more than just the sun would rise here as the girls were going through basic training.

This is where Rocky fit in. Since he had some experience as a masseuse from his Air Force days, Phil chose him to handpick and teach the good looking "pupils" the tricks of the trade. Rocky had the ideal job of interviewing the gals and then having them apply their hand and finger techniques on him. He took no money for his services but did receive sexual favors along the way.

In his spare time Rocky volunteered to do a photoset with the University of Wisconsin's Art Department by posing nude. One of his "back shots" was used for an advertisement for the Rising Sun in a Madison newspaper, enabling the owner to lure in clientele to the uptown massage parlor. Genie's Magic Touch was Phil Barrot's second downtown Madison parlor to come into play, and a third one opened its doors on the west side sometime later.

Rocky decided it was time to move into his own one-bedroom apartment. Whispering Oaks was located on the Beltline in Madison across from the Coliseum. He severed his relationship with Kerry, which didn't go over very well with her, and then gave the front door key to his castle to his blonde tootsie. After a few months, Ruby became highly possessive in nature and somewhat tiresome to be around. They had a huge fight and a bad break-up. Rocky confiscated his apartment key and was a free soul once again.

Still enjoying the handful of pleasurable benefits from the massage parlor life, Rocky continued working for Phil Barrot. One afternoon he walked into one of the heavy traffic parlors and asked for one of their special services from the menu. When the body massage was completed, he tried to coax the chosen masseuse into going a few steps further. "What would it take for us to go around the world? How about fifty smackers more?" This honest employee just happened to deny his request, and she was safe for the time being. Rocky's job was to test out Phil's girls to see if they would put out or not. If they were lured in, the Man would have to drop a dime on them, and they would be fired on the spot. There were a handful of undercover cops nonchalantly sneaking around. If the Madison cops had their way, these massage parlors would be blown to shreds by moving tanks. For the love of money, Phil did not want to get shut down.

A movie came to Rocky's mind that was on the tube a while back about a playboy stalking the college campus where he was enrolled. This guy was on the lookout to bang every girl in sight.

Some nights Mr. Studly had two different girls in one night. He kept a record on his calendar of all of the sexual performances.

One night an art show was put on at the college by some of the professors, and many of the sorority girls attended. They began conversing about this super stud on campus and all of his activities, and eventually they put two and two together and figured out what he was up to.

The babes came up with a master plan. A couple of nights later the sorority sisters caught this sex maniac by the balls, so to speak, chained his hands and feet, gagged him with a putrid-smelling sock and Scotch tape, and forced him all the way up into the third floor attic of a sorority house. The overpowered male was dominated by a large handful of wild, sex-crazed women! They'd lured him up there to stroke and wear him down to a frazzle. When his fraternity brothers knew that Mr. Studly could not take one ounce more, he was finally rescued from the leather-and-laced female mob bosses. Studly became a heroic legend in his own time who was never forgotten.

After seeing that movie, Rocky started going out to the Left Guard restaurant in Madison, a very hot pickup joint to get girls. He picked up a different gal each night for thirty nights straight and also put a notch on his own calendar like Mr. Studly in the movie. He had no respect for women after his first marriage.

After thirty nights, Rocky received a signal from a higher psychic creature in another universe. It must have been the Lord who told Rocky to cool his jets for a while and to start thinking about his immediate future. To have an eternal glowing future with the best humans on earth, he would have to prove that he was worthy in the light of the Father and gain his respect.

After this experience, Rocky decided that this kind of life was one that he did not want to lead. His instinct was to phone Ruby once again for a date. She accepted, and they went out for a memorable dinner and spent a romantic evening together by the fireplace, watching each other's naked shadows in the flickering dim light. It was at Ruby's log cabin home that Rocky scored once again. He scored his second wife, knowing that he was drug-free and in desperate need of changing his life.

The couple was married, and they took on the log cabin home as their residency. Ruby was a very attractive brown-eyed girl who wore excessive makeup. When it came to the bedroom, Ruby was the aggressor, but with everything else, Rocky was in total control.

In 1975, while still married to Ruby, Rocky started lifting heavily again. He acquired a mind-boggling idea: what if he could adjust his weight to precisely 220 pounds? The Olympic year was coming up in 1976 with a new weight category of 220 pounds, and just the clean and jerk plus the snatch lift would be presented. By training hard and being on the correct diet for his body, his goal was now to qualify for this competition-class weight drug-free!

In the 242-pound category Rocky's best clean and jerk was 405 pounds, and his top snatch lift was 305. When his bodyweight was exactly 220 pounds, his best clean and jerk was recorded at 370, with a snatch at a remarkable 270 pounds. Although he was twenty-two pounds lighter, Rocky was only thirty-five pounds away from his heavier bodyweight scores.

On the night of the state championship competition in Milwaukee, the huge muscular man's foot got caught in the platform, causing his knee to buckle and turn out during his performance. His quadriceps was ripped off of his knee, along with three-quarters of the patella tendon. Rocky could not get up. The massive weight from the barbell just missed striking him. His quad retracted twelve inches up from the knee, leaving a noticeable gap in the leg. As Rocky was being lifted onto a stretcher, Ruby ran over by the platform and yelled out, "That was a stupid thing to do. How am I going to get home now? You know I don't know how to drive in Milwaukee."

Rocky slowly turned his neck in Ruby's direction and calmly said, "You're such a gem." He was hauled off in a station wagon to a local hospital in Milwaukee. Doctor David Mellencamp was the orthopedic surgeon on duty, and he was also the head physician at the Milwaukee hospital. After studying the x-rays, the surgeon explained that this was an unbelievable freak accident. He only knew of one other similar tear like this, which happened to a professional basketball player. A five-hour operation was performed as the skilled surgeon stitched the quadriceps back into the knee area using a precision technique. Later, a cast that stretched from the ankle to the hip anchored his leg in place. Within the next ten days a staph infection penetrated into the skin, which in turn caused severe swelling. The cast was split down the middle and removed, and Rocky was put on intravenous antibiotics.

Doctor Mellencamp later gave Rocky the news that he did not want to hear: "Your weightlifting career is over." Rocky couldn't believe it. He'd just wanted to prove to himself and anyone else who was following his career that he was going to be one of the best Olympic champions who had ever lived—DRUG FREE. Now he felt that GOD took this chance away from him for a second time. In 1964 it was that painful arm injury, and now the damaged leg accident would prevent him from any foreseeable chance of competing in the Olympics. In his mind, God was deeply at fault.

The suffering, broken-down ego of this massive weightlifter was put at a standstill while his unstable body lay flat on its backbone at the hospital for a total of ten days. When his pain killers wore off, the mind had more than enough time to think, sometimes irrationally.

"You were always my Gipper, my savior, when I was growing up. Now you put a stop to my growing. I'm at a turning point in my life. You've taken away all of my ambitions and desires. You have denied me the right to be a champion. Now I know what sports writers mean when they talk about the agony of defeat. After praying to you for all these years, look where it has gotten me. My life is over. What do I do now—play a fiddle out on the street corner?

"I know that I've been so wrapped up in lifting again, and I haven't been home much or give much thought about my work efforts. Ruby really hates when I'm gone because she always wants to be the center of attention. Maybe that's why she hasn't called me and only came to see me once so far. She thinks that I'm a jerk!

"Oh, what the hell. My life will get better someday. I can't feel sorry for myself anymore. I will not let depression set in to threaten me. For a few seconds there my thoughts were going into a different direction. What if the devil has more power than my Gipper? Maybe that evil son-of-a-bitch is controlling my life!"

After the agonizing accident, Rocky had Ruby drive him around on the job in his territory to once again have a relationship with his customers. It was hard to get in and out of their vehicle with a full-length cast on. Mickey, Ruby's son from a previous marriage, would go along to swim in the nearby in-ground heated pools. It almost seemed like Ruby was the spokesperson on the job, as she created much attention by wearing her red bikini out in the sun in front of Rocky's clients.

Because of his latest injuries, Rocky thought that he would cool his jets for a while and coach a power lifting team. There was a group of high school kids from Spring Grove who knew of Norman Rauch and would give an arm and a leg to be on his team. All Rocky wanted was for them to give their best possible efforts toward the sport. After a period of hard-training workouts, the coach took his kids to a power lifting championship. While spending the first night in a hotel room, one of the boys snuck out and got himself liquored up by using a fake ID. The kid started to get the hot flashes when he arrived back in the room. His head started to spin like a skater on ice, and he started to "flash" on everything in sight. Heave-ho! The smell alone was bad enough to make you want to gag.

The next evening, the boys told Rocky they were also interested in bodybuilding. Rocky started to tell them a little bit about his history and showed them a couple of vein-popping poses. For the time being he knew that he could at least keep his muscular framework in great shape. The kids went on to place second in the competition, and photographs were inserted into the local newspapers with them all wearing Pebble Valley t-shirts.

Between the puking stories and Rocky prancing around in his underwear, the events were taken slightly out of context. When the principal received wind of this behavior, he felt that it was his duty to call each and every parent. The next day there were mothers and fathers flocking into the high school like a herd of sheep.

"What do you mean my boy was involved in a beer-chugging contest while the fag coach stripped down in front of our boys?" yelled one of the kids' parents.

"It didn't quite happen in that manner, madam," explained the principal. With the way kids like to brag, gossip, and stretch the truth, it's no wonder that their parents were on the warpath. There was finally a meeting with the principal, Rocky, and the parents.

"If any of this untruthful gossip leaks out into the newspapers," said Rocky angrily, "I will pursue this to the highest level, and each and every one of you will be sitting across from a jury in a court of law." This was Rocky's opening statement. "This major happening took place because of the effort and hard work that your boys and I put into it. And no, I was not exposing myself to your kids in the hotel room. I know this was not part of any high school program." This is what also frosted the wrestling and football coaches.

They made a comment to the principal later on in the day, "What is this crap all about? This guy isn't even connected with our school!"

Rocky had been trying to do something good for the kids and felt that he was being blacklisted by the community, but all that excitement was actually put on the back burner after he spoke his peace. He was still training with the boys when one night he wrapped his bad leg, put on a lifting belt, and squatted 400 pounds with all the weight on his good leg. That was very amazing for the kids to witness. He was also bench pressing around 350 pounds and dead lifting 500 pounds at the bodyweight of 220 pounds.

The huge powerful man decided to enter the Wisconsin State Power Lifting Championship just one year after his last leg accident. A monster of a guy by the first name of Billy was the only other lifter in his weight class. Billy started the competition with a startling weight of 600 pounds and missed his first squat attempt. Billy actually missed the next two lifts and bombed out. All Rocky had to do was to make one lift out of the three for the three different categories. He won this challenge with a bad leg. People thought he was crazy in the first place for even thinking about entering this competition. His doctors weren't even notified. He assumed that was the last power lifting contest he would ever be involved in. He just wanted to prove that he still had it in him to be a champion.

Being out on the road a lot for his job, Norman would sometimes get a little homesick and call his wife Ruby. One night he made three or four calls until he finally reached her at around three o'clock in the morning. "I was trying to get a hold of you," said Norman. "Where have you been all this time?"

"I went to a Tup…Tupperware party," stuttered Ruby.

"Tupperware parties do not last until three in the morning," answered her husband.

"I know, but it was also a girls' night out…for drinks," said Ruby.

"But nothing stays open that late in our vicinity," stated Rocky.

"We all went out to the greasy spoon for coffee," Ruby said with a yawn.

"You don't like coffee," stated her husband. "Tell me right now what's going on."

"Nothing. Nothing at all," she said before the telephone receiver bounced off of the carpet and the line went dead.

Rocky knew that there was something going on but did not want to reveal it to his ego. He wanted to prove to himself that she had no reason to cheat on someone who supported her like he did, so he arrived home one night in the wee hours of the morning and sat in the kitchen with the lights off.

Ruby slightly staggered into the room and flipped on the light switch, "What the hell are you doing sitting here in the dark? Checking up on me?" She had Mickey in her arms, and he rubbed the sleep out of his eyes and started to cry. Ruby turned around and headed for the child's bedroom.

Rocky said to himself in a low tone, "She looks as if she just got sucked through a knothole backwards."

Ruby entered the kitchen with a sense of authority and shouted, "Mr. Rauch, I'll make you a deal that no man could ever refuse. I know that you're thinking that I've been cheating on you, so let's just say that we go our separate ways when you are out of town. You can do whatever you want, and I'll do the same. Then when you are home I'll cook for you and do your dirty laundry. We'll stay married. How does that sound?"

"What if you get pregnant?" asked Rocky.

"That won't ever happen," said Ruby, "I'd be careful, and you know I would never want to lose this shape." Norman had a vasectomy performed after having two children from his previous marriage. Having more children at the time was not his idea of having fun.

"This marriage is over," shouted Rocky. Ruby stormed across the kitchen and started to throw a temper tantrum, and that's not all she threw. She slid a long-handled butcher knife out of its wooden rack and tossed it directly at Rocky's chest. If the knife would have turned one more time the blade would have stuck.

Seconds before this charade, Rocky had wanted to just carry her off into the bedroom and prove to himself that she was having sex with another man, but now he had completely lost it. He picked her up and slammed her across the room and through the bathroom door. Having no sense of balance, Ruby conked her head and landed in the porcelain tub. She lay there for a long while. Rocky thought he had killed her. This was the very first time he had ever laid hands on a woman.

Once he knew that she was all right, Rocky yelled, "If you climb out of that bathtub, I will rip your head off! Now listen up. I will put $100 in a checking account and $100 in a savings account. The last three payments will be made on your car, and the half side of beef will be left in the freezer for you. I will be contacting my attorney tomorrow and filing for a divorce. Any questions yet?" Rocky reached for Ruby's pocket book, whipped out all the credit cards, and shoved them into his trousers. "Now do yourself a favor and go out and get a job before your money runs out and you starve to death. I'll have a moving truck here within five days. I'm taking out of this house exactly what I first came in with."

CHAPTER 6
OUT WITH THE OLD AND IN WITH THE NEW

Out on his road to freedom, Rocky focused his thoughts on the person he was going to miss the most. Rocky was all alone now and didn't have the slightest clue where he was going or what he was going to do, and he couldn't help but think about a kid he had become attached to.

Mickey had been short and fat when he first hooked up with Ruby. He didn't look right from the start. Rocky always thought there was something wrong with him and he would never grow. Mickey was undersized for his age, but Ruby didn't pay much attention to my way of thinking and said that her kid would sprout up like a bean stock someday.

He didn't grow for the longest time. Rocky remembered making an appointment to have his mother take him to the children's department of the University of Wisconsin Hospital. The specialists diagnosed him with the problem of having an inactive thyroid. They put him on special medicine and told them to bring Mickey in every three weeks for another examination. One of the doctors thanked Rocky for being concerned and bringing the kid in for a checkup. If he hadn't, the boy would have been the size of a midget for the rest of his life.

Rocky told Ruby to continue to take her son in for checkups for the rest of his life. He hoped Mickey would understand someday what he did for him, and he hoped that Mickey would always remember him as a person to look up to. Maybe he would never see the boy again. Who knew? He realized he could take a liking to kids if he didn't have to spend a whole lot of time taking care of them.

The vehicle that Norman Rauch was subconsciously driving piloted him right into the Huffman House parking lot in Milwaukee. This joint was sort of a pickup place if you wanted something from a person of the opposite sex. Nonchalantly, Norman walked toward one of the back booths and ordered an orange juice on the rocks from the waitress. His mind started to wander once again, thinking about how he could have ever gotten mixed up in another unfavorable marriage.

"I don't have the slightest idea where I'm going to rest my head tonight," thought Rocky. A blonde woman with a male companion chasing after her walked by his table and made eye contact with a glowing, fresh smile before walking out the front door.

"Here's your straight orange juice on ice," stated the hot waitress. "You sure I can't freshen that drink up for you with something that could make you feel more relaxed?"

"I don't think that you are quite tiny enough to fit into my glass," snickered Rocky, "but keep working on that tight ass of yours."

"You silly boy," said the waitress as she walked away, looking for another way to make a good tip.

Approximately fifteen minutes later, the same blonde who had made eye contact with Rocky before sat down in the booth right across from him and said, "Excuse me, buddy. May I sit down here with you?"

"It looks to me like you already have," said Rocky staring at her cleavage.

"I hardly ever am so forward to ask this," stated the sweet-smelling blonde, "but it looks to me like you are a little bit under the weather. I feel that you might just need some company."

"Well, I guess you're right," agreed Rocky. "I do have a few problems going on in my life right now."

"You know, I have a problem also," interrupted the pretty lady. "I was trying to celebrate a job promotion with my married friend that walked out on me. Mr. Jerkoff had to go home to wifey dear and left me all by my lonesome. It was supposed to be a special night for me."

"Married friend, eh?" chuckled Rocky. "What's that all about, if you don't mind me asking?"

"Well, I believe it's safer to go out with married guys," explained the blonde. "He pays for most of the rent on my apartment. But I guess anymore he only comes around when he wants to get laid. I feel like I'm being used."

"You asked for it in more ways than one," said Rocky.

"What's your problem?" asked the blonde. "And by the way, my friends all call me Sapphire. What may I call you?"

"Not another gem," thought Norman. Aloud, he said, "My friends all call me the Real Rocky. I am still in a marriage that's for the birds. Actually, I left her today for good, and right at the moment I have no particular place to go."

"It looks like we're sort of in the same boat, Mr. Real Rocky," stated Sapphire.

"For now, I know of a place right around the corner called the Left Guard," explained Rocky. "A friend of mine from the Green Bay Packers has a partnership there. May I escort you, my dear?"

"I would be honored, Real Rocky," said Sapphire, latching on to his shoulder muscles.

The young, good-looking couple conversed about their backgrounds and some everyday problems while still flirting with each other with minor caressing at the Left Guard. But it wasn't long before this gem was wasted and noticeably slurring her speech. It was getting late, and Rocky had to work the next morning. "Where do you live, and how did you get into this neighborhood?" asked Rocky.

"I don't live that fa…far away, and my car is parked back at the Huff…Huffman House," stated Sapphire.

Rocky spoke up, "You're not driving home. I'll give you a ride."

"Well, then how am I supposed to get to my ride tomorrow, Mr. Big Shot?" asked Sapphire.

"That's a good question," answered Rocky. "How about if I pick you up in the morning so you can get your car?"

"Bet…better idea," slurred the inebriated young blonde. "You can spend the night with me." Rocky took advantage of the situation and woke up naked the next morning with Sapphire hanging all over him.

During breakfast at the kitchenette table Rocky broke the ice, "So I don't have to waste money on a motel room, do you think I could stay here another night while I look for a cheap place to rent?"

"Oh, sure, but I won't be home until 7:00 p.m.," answered Sapphire. After breakfast she got dressed, put her makeup on in a flash, and handed Rocky the front door key to her apartment and was on her way. "See you later on tonight, big boy." She didn't even think to ask Rocky what his last name was.

All day at work Sapphire visualized her apartment being wiped out and coming home to a bare living room and bedroom, with the stud long gone. How would she explain this to the cops? She knew nothing about the guy that she just had a one-night stand with.

Being the nice guy that he was, Rocky picked up a bottle of wine and a couple of steaks on his way back from West Bend, where he'd worked that day. He was going to surprise his new sex partner with a home-cooked meal. When she arrived at her apartment that evening, Sapphire was very relieved to see all the furniture and stereo equipment still intact. Even her white poodle Mitchie was at the front door to greet her with a smile and a friendly howl.

"Let's sing along with Mitch," chuckled Rocky.

"Oh, what a darling you are," said Sapphire. "You even have the table set with candles flickering. What is that succulent aroma that I smell?"

Since Rocky's new mate was completely sober, he had a serious talk with her over a delicious meal. "I really have nowhere to hang my hat, and I'm getting a little desperate about finding a place to stay."

"Oh, honey, you could always live here with me," said Sapphire.

"This is what I'm afraid of," answered Norm. "I'll have to think about this for a while."

"Or you could stay in another apartment in this complex," stated the young blonde, licking her bluish lipstick.

"You're such a tease," said Norman, "but my financial situation is not very stable at the moment."

The next day Rocky put a lot of thought into what he was going to do over the weekend that was coming up. He decided that he would go up to Elkhart Lake for the races on his Harley and live in a tent. He invited Sapphire. Rocky set up his tent and equipment in her yard to make sure everything was in order. Of course, one thing led to another and they never did get off the ground on that expensive Harley. Instead, they took the motorcycle over to her parents' house to put in storage, as the life expectancy of a brand new Harley on the streets of Milwaukee was approximately three minutes. Sapphire's mom and dad thought that Rocky was a free-loader. A month later Sapphire and Rocky rented a moving truck to haul all of his belongings back to her apartment.

Rocky and his attorney strolled one step ahead of Ruby as they climbed the courthouse front steps and entered through the huge front doors. They were all in a hurry to get this divorce court day over with, except for the raving judge. "You people don't have a case here. There must be a cause or a ground for choice or action. A lot of fighting and screaming just doesn't cut the mustard. Even I can scream! Where did you pass your bar exam, counselor—down at the local tavern? You're all wasting my time. Get out of my courtroom. Next case, bailiff."

They all stopped at the nearest greasy spoon for coffee. "We need something better than incompatibility, my friends," said the lawyer. "Any suggestions?"

"How about this?" answered Norman. "Ruby, remember the night when we did a bit more than just argue? You tried your damnedest to put a butcher knife through my heart, and I got pissed and threw you through two rooms into the bathtub. You want to hear more?"

"Hey, that's good. No, that's great!" exclaimed Rocky's attorney. "That's your ticket to freedom. Let's go back and see Mr. Hardass Judge." They waited three hours for the same judge to hear their case once again. He reluctantly accepted this story after polygraph testing and told the now-divorced couple that they were both crazy.

At the base of the courthouse concrete steps, Ruby asked Norman for $5 so she could find some transportation home. He just laughed and gave her a fin out of his wallet. The attorney looked over at Rocky and said, "You should have made her do tricks for it."

Another four or five weeks zoomed by when Sapphire and Rocky decided to rent a larger apartment in the same complex. He would give her his paycheck every week, and she would pay all the bills and distribute the remaining cash for toys that they both wanted. They lived together for around three years. It wasn't until the third year that Rocky started to work out again, just to keep in shape.

Sapphire was a hardcore drinker. If she was drinking on a particular day, she would go for all the gusto, no stopping along the way. This bothered Rocky immensely because he was brought up with parents who both drank, sometimes rather heavily.

Eventually they moved into a duplex together and got married. From time to time Rocky would remember what Sapphire had told him after a year of living together. She said that it would be one giant step for this gal to even think about marriage again. It had something to do with an ex-husband who received a big promotion and then ran off with his secretary. He filed for a divorce and pretty much got everything. She said to Rocky once, "If I ever get married again and that guy is untrue to me, I will take that joker to the cleaners, lock, stock, and barrel. I'll rake him over the coals if I have to."

The happily married couple ended up buying a nice home in Madison. Rocky's office for the pump company was there. Sapphire did not want to give up her position as a field representative for the Milwaukee Blood Center, so she would commute back and forth. During the week, Sapphire stayed with her mother after her parents broke up. Her mother also had a drinking problem. The couple were together on weekends, but Rocky had complete control of the house during the week.

One night after work, Rocky put a supreme deep dish pizza in the oven and then sat down in his favorite chair and let his mind wander.

Boy, the time that I went to that motorcycle show in Madison with my friend Randy was certainly a blast. I remember when I first had my bike custom-painted and turned it into a street rod. That weekend I saw my polished Harley glimmering in the sunlight along next to a thousand other cycles of all different shapes and sizes. The Home Town Ryders bike club was there with their many choppers and beer steins on display. It was definitely a party in the city for three exciting days.

The very first bike that I paid $750 for was a real prize. The guy at the shop had to show me how to steer the damn thing around the circular-drive blacktop. I first learned on a piece of Jap crap how to ride, and I got my temporary bike permit out of the deal. I guess that I should think of it more as a rice-burner from heaven. One night after work I drove that small 360 past the Harley shop and did a double take. The most beautiful bikes that I had ever seen were on display on the showroom floor.

I parked my bike around the back where nobody could see me getting off of it and took a stroll inside of heaven's gates to see the headlights of a 1200 Superglide staring me right in the face. "Now that's a bike," I remember saying to one of the salesmen.

A couple of days later I traded off my rice-burning scooter for exactly what I paid for it and drove that real machine out of the Harley showroom. The day that I went in to take my written and driving test to get my license, there were people staring out of the state office building windows. Then a crowd formed in the parking lot. I remember one of the State Examiners saying that they didn't even know if their road course could even handle a motorcycle of that size. A 1200 Superglide is like a full dresser but without the side trimmings. This giant machine could glide around the barricades with ease, and I had no trouble making it perform for the officials to be granted a permanent motorcycle license.

All of a sudden Rocky lost his train of thought because he could smell something burning in the kitchen. "Oh, shit! My pizza's probably burning in the oven while I'm sitting here like a dope reminiscing about the past." He was able to salvage most of the overcooked pizza, and he sat down again with a couple of slices and a frosted beer mug.

When I would touch the motorcycle handlebars with the engine purring like a mountain lion, I would get the same rush as when I would first latch onto a bar with massive weights on both ends in a competition. It was the most fantastic feeling anyone could ever have. It was like you just had to conquer the bar and be a master of the world around you.

A couple of weeks after the bike show, I remember calling on one of my customers when a truck pulled up with a load for them. A plain-looking guy with glasses hopped down from his rig and gave me the once-over. His hair was not that long but not real short either. He had a pack of smokes rolled up in his t-shirt sleeve, but I didn't see any noticeable tattoos. This cat was more of a greaser type of guy. He asked me if I was up at the last bike show in Madison and if my name was Rocky. I answered, "You bet," to both questions and we started talking. The guy said that he introduced himself to me at the show as A.B.

Well, I found out that this normal-looking nice guy was the president of the well-known Home Town Ryders bike club. A.B. wanted me to go up and check out his motorcycle club sometime and said that he would sponsor me. At the time Sapphire and I lived in Milwaukee, and I told A.B. that it would be hard to be in a bike club out of Madison with my schedule and everything, but I would certainly think about it. It wasn't too much longer after seeing A.B. again that Sapphire and I moved to Madison so I could be closer to my work office. Of course, I gave A.B. a call.

Rocky decided to go to a meeting at the club house of the Home Town Ryders bike club as a guest of A.B. and thought seriously about becoming a member. You couldn't just strut right in and say that you want to ride your chopper in their bike gang. It didn't work like that. If the officials and regular members thought that you were a good candidate, they would consider you as a prospect for a period of time until they thought you were ready. A series of random and scheduled initiation exercises were also on the agenda. It was similar to being a recruit in the army, but with more riding than marching.

Rocky eventually became a full-fledged member of the Home Town Ryders bike Club. A B. did give him one good piece of information. If you were given a direct order to do something, you could always turn around and challenge that member during your probationary period. Let's say Tiny told you to get down in the dirt and give him fifty push-ups, the candidate could politely say, "Please show me how it's done." If Tiny could not do the full fifty repetitions himself, then the recruit wouldn't have to take that order.

Another part of the training was to be able to memorize every member's real birth name and also all of their nicknames. There were approximately forty-five group members at the time, which made this process a big challenge.

The Home Town Ryders bike club was a very tight network, and once you made it in, you became a member for life. You could never just walk out on them, but you could be evicted for breaking a club rule. They taught you from the start to put your life on the line for your fellow brothers. The club members got along with most other races in the outside world, except for the rednecks. That was one group that they couldn't tolerate.

They had a good relationship with the Madison Police Department. One of the club rules was never to wheel and deal drugs of any kind, but some of the boys had their own preference when it came to using drugs. Snorting coke was a great rush, along with speed to get the body motivated. A rolled zigzag joint being passed around the campfire was also a pleasurable way of relaxing the mind.

The club members all had special duties to perform, including donating blood to the Red Cross. There was a blood chairman in charge of the blood drives, and some of the more experienced bikers strutted around with thirty or more blood donation pins attached to their chests. Some of the cops on the police force would hang around with the Home Town Ryders at the clubhouse after hours. They were always welcome. The bike members put on quite of few fundraisers, always for a worthy cause.

The July Fourth outdoor bash was coming up soon, and Rocky was elected to find and set up two huge rotisseries and purchase two hindquarters of beef. The bike club rented a couple of acres of land outside of Madison. Plans were voted on to set up a giant tent and hire a well-known band, and of course strippers would be needed for this fun-filled event of bikers coming from all over the country.

Since Rocky was put in charge of organizing all of the food, he had to start this giant feast preparation a couple of days in advance. Between 800 and 1,000 bikers rode in and happily paid the price of $25 a plate for food with entertainment included. It was like an old Wild West show, except choppers were used to carry the riders instead of horses, and M-80s and bottle rockets were fired into the air instead of six-shooters. The fireworks they shot off sounded more like canons being shot off for a 21-gun salute.

The next morning Rocky and his helpers cooked over 2,000 eggs for breakfast. He glanced at bikers coming through the outdoor cafeteria-style line of all shapes and sizes. One guy had a bone and rings through his nose, at least five pierced earrings, and tattoos everywhere.

This kind of Fourth of July party was put on every year to make money for the club. This event happened to be one of the better bashes ever put on by the club, so Rocky was chosen to receive the How'd Ya Award. This was quite an honor to be given to a prospect of the Home Town Ryders bike club for doing a great job for fellow Americans.

That evening the president of the Madison club got up on a platform inside the erected tent and boasted, "Our man of the hour, Mr. Rocky Rauch, has been selected to win his first major award as a prospect of our chapter." Rocky was presented with this award while a well-respected song played in the background. The last line of the song lyrics went something like this, "How'd ya like to kiss my ass?" Rocky also received, with dignity, a pat on the back (and sometimes on the ass) by over 800 bikers of every nationality. The Italians especially knew how to speak with their hands.

After being a prospect for two months, Rocky thought that it should be about time that he became a member. The grunts had to wear their colors on their vests with the word PROSPECT on the bottom rocker. When you became a full-fledged member, the top rocker of your colors would be filled in with Home Town Ryders and a picture of the capitol building would be displayed in the middle. The bottom rocker would then be changed to MADISON, WISCONSIN, to take the place of PROSPECT. Not all prospects became members. If you didn't do what you were told to do or if other members didn't like you, then you weren't voted in.

Rocky went to a club meeting one night at around 7:00 and was told that he would become a member if he passed the initiation process that was going to take place immediately. The leaders in charge ordered him to remove his shirt so that they could paint his torso green, like the Incredible Hulk. Then he was told to climb on his Harley with a passenger of their choice. His partner for the evening was an inflatable doll. The plan was for Rocky to visit five different taverns in a certain period of time.

While on the road for a brief period with two plastic nipples poking him in the backside, he located his first tavern. He was to pick out an object that didn't look like it should really be there and carry it with him and his date. A big two-foot log about ten inches in diameter was close to the entranceway of the tavern, so Rocky picked it up with one hand while hanging onto his mate for the time being. There were a few odd stares being shot in his direction, as Rocky indispensably walked into the bar with a log and his hog. He propped up his date on the bar stool next to him and proceeded to order two shots of Jack Daniels. The bartender snickered, "I suppose one of these is for your playmate," as she set one shot in front of Rocky and one in front of his doll.

Just about that time two members of the Home Town Ryders bike club followed him into the tavern and started to take photographs, so Rocky followed the orders given to him and scampered back outside with the doll to find the next bar on his own accord.

At the next tavern Rocky shouted over the music to the bartender, "May I please have two shots of Jack, one for me and one for my girlfriend?" He was told to say that at each bar.

The guy on the other side of Rocky's playmate, who was about three sheets to the wind, stammered to the bartender, "Is that guy on the other side of his naked girlfriend real…really green, or is that my mind pl…playing tricks on me?"

The bartender chuckled, "That's really the Incredible Hulk with a beautiful naked lady."

The drunk admitted, "I think maybe I had just a wee bit too mu…much to drink. I'm going home now. See…see you." The bartender and Rocky had a good laugh over that one.

After Rocky found the last three taverns and accumulated ten chips for ordering ten shots, he had one last thing on the agenda to do before going back to the shop. He had to bring his date back fully dressed. Now where was he going to find clothes for a naked plastic doll at 7:30 at night?

Rocky had only a total of one hour to complete this entire fun-filled adventure, or he would fail his initiation. So he went to the nearest Goodwill bin to see what good fortunes could bring him. The chest of junk was locked, but Rocky jiggled the lock and was able to reach into the opening. He pulled out the most awful-looking black dress that fit his naked date. Amazing!

He rode like the wind back to the Wisconsin Hut bar, where he had to report back. The back door where the pool sharks hung out was flung open, and Rocky threw down his now-dressed doll on the nearest pool table. The two-foot log crashed to the ground, and the ten drink chips went flying. "I made it with flying colors!" exclaimed the latest member of the club.

None of the guys could believe their eyes when they saw Rocky rush through that door with about seven minutes to spare. As the president of the Home Town Ryders fitted the new member with his tailor-made vest and colors, the guys commended him while pouring pitchers of beer over his head and down into the front side of his leather skins. The Home Town Ryders club house was directly in back of the Wisconsin Hut where Rocky had to meet his real date for the evening. You might say that Rocky got lucky twice on that fantastic clear, starry night.

Rocky's third gem, Sapphire, was not accustomed to being part of such an opinionated clique of bike-crazed non-conformists. She kept saying that she couldn't believe that this biker's world was part of her everyday living. Although Rocky was allowed to go up to Black River Falls to sponsor his very own prospect on a long Memorial Day weekend. Sapphire decided to tag along and drive their van and trailer in case a motorcycle went out of commission and needed to be hauled to a place of repair. There was going to be a campout at one of the club members' farmlands.

That evening most of the boys wanted to go into town and raise a ruckus. Using his head, Rocky said that would not be a very cool idea because the members didn't know the area very well. They all went anyway, including the prospect, because he didn't have much of a choice in the matter. The boys had a ball and got juiced to the gills. On the way back to the campgrounds later on, a deer ran out in front of the bike convoy and spoiled their evening. The prospect in the back of the pack ran into the Harley directly in front of him because his reaction time was on a delayed timer due to alcohol. The biker in front inherited a broken arm, and his lady received a mind-boggling concussion, but the prospect went into a coma from head injuries and never recovered. Rocky felt bad at the funeral because the kid was only twenty years old, and he never got the chance to live his life to its fullest.

His wife supported Rocky for over three years with the Home Town Ryders bike club. There were many good times and also some bad times. He gradually went back into the art of bodybuilding, and some of the bikers even drove a motorhome into Chicago to watch him perform in The American competition. As a dedicated member, Rocky became very close to all of the other club member brothers.

In 1982, something terrible happened that stirred up a bit of trouble for the Home Town Ryders biker organization. There was a big party held in Madison. It was put on by another bike gang that was associated with the Milwaukee Inlaws, which just happened to be a sister-chapter club to the infamous California Heaven's Angels. Benny Klove, one of the Home Town Ryders club enforcers, got himself pretty well snookered up and decided to argue over something petty. Someone at that moment with a fidgety trigger finger blew poor Benny's brains out all over the floor in front of him. It was a gang-style killing that was projected over the National Wire Service the next day. On a Sunday morning, Rocky received a call to be at a special meeting at their club house by ten o-clock sharp. Everyone was warned to beware of a war between the motorcycle rivalries.

Before he went to the important meeting of the chapter members, Rocky received a call from his boss, Gill Hanson. "I heard that there was a shooting that involved the club that you are a member of."

"Yeah, Gill, you heard right," stated Rocky.

"Well, I'm going to give you two choices," insisted Gill. "I know you've worked for me for a long time, and you are like family. But you can't represent my company with those kind of credentials hanging over your head. You can either work for my company or be a Home Town Ryder, but you can't do both. You have to make one of the choices now. What's your decision going to be? You only have five more seconds of my time, Mr. Rauch."

"I want to work for you, Gill," Rocky expressed immediately.

So after that telephone call, Rocky hurriedly rode over to the Home Town Ryders clubhouse for the ten o'clock meeting. The members were all told to be sharp and on their guard at all times. They were to be on the lookout for anything out of the ordinary going on, any foul play or tampering of any kind with their belongings.

The following week, everyone attended the funeral procession for Benny, the club enforcer. There was always a huge gathering of all the brothers and friends when someone passed away. Then on Monday of the next week, Rocky attended one of their regular meetings to bring up something of importance in front of the officers and members.

"The owner and boss of my company has given me the ultimatum to either be a Home Town Ryder or to keep my job," explained Rocky. "And I can't afford to lose that paycheck, so I am resigning as a member of the Home Town Ryders bike club organization. It was my decision to make, but I want everyone here to know that I was forced into this situation."

"On behalf of the Home Town Ryders, we do not want to inactivate you and put you out of the club," announced the president as he took the floor. "We would like to pronounce you as an inactive member for the rest of your natural life. That way you can still wear your colors high with honor and dignity. We will leave you in good standings, and you'll always be a brother."

The vote was unanimous.

CHAPTER 7
THE LUSH AGAINST HIS RUSH

Just the thought of Rocky leaving the bike club put Sapphire's mind to rest for the time being. She eventually persuaded her husband to purchase a split-level ranch style house closer to the Milwaukee area. Rocky really didn't like this idea but went along with it to fulfill one of her dreams. Without the brotherhood of the Home Town Ryders to occupy his time, Rocky felt empty and restless inside. So once again, he seriously started to train for another bodybuilding championship. Sapphire did not understand his compulsive behaviors any more than any of his other wives did. The more time he devoted to his training, the more she withdrew into her own addictive behavior, guzzling flasks of Rhine wine. When she wasn't working, she was drinking. Sapphire reached her record high of eight gallons per week, and of course her husband spent most of his free time in the gym. The arguing between them steadily escalated until their marriage was simply drowning.

Around every fourth week Rocky would cover the job market in Milwaukee, so he and his wife would stay together in a motel. It was usually a drag, with a lot of arguments and fighting. Rocky would get off work at around six o'clock and go straight to the gym for an hour and a half workout session. Depending on how much bullshitting took place, he would make it back to the motel in the neighborhood of eight o'clock to take his wife out for a meal. This really bugged Sapphire. She thought that she was always competing with his weight training.

In 1982, at the ripe age of forty, Rocky trained very hard for the upcoming Mr. Wisconsin Over 35 Championship. He was disappointed when he only took home the title of runner-up in the competition. Not one to be dissuaded, the muscular giant set his crosshairs on the Mr. America Over 40 contest. With approximately six months to get into superior shape before the national championship, Rocky was easily persuaded to upgrade his chances of winning by taking steroids. Some of the boys in the gym were saying, "You need to get with it, Rocky. You need to get on the sauce."

It had been eleven years since the big man had taken Dianabol, and programs in the steroid world were changing dramatically. Rocky was willing to take the advice of other serious weightlifters where he worked out. Most of these guys knew a lot about the more complex combinations of steroids that had become available. They knew most everything, except for the fact that they could totally destroy your immune system, which could cause you to keel over and drop dead.

All the aging ex-champion could think about was his obsession of winning, and there was no doubt in his mind that all of his fellow competitors were on the sauce. Rocky conveniently emptied his brain cells of past thoughts of a deteriorated liver, a low white blood count, and numerous raging skin boils. Using steroids had become the norm in this world of bodybuilding. In his mind, without this drug, he would have no chance of winning any more state or national competition titles.

The more modern anabolic steroid programs consisted of taking the oral drugs and also injections. Durabolin, Anavar, Anadrol Primobolan, and Winstrol, to name a few, were the group that Rocky quickly familiarized himself with. He learned how much of each one to take and the correct pronunciations of the names as well. There was never a problem with getting a hold of this type of drug. Numerous guys in the gym were selling them, and doctors in the Milwaukee area were prescribing them. Rocky was referred to a physician who, for a $25 fee, would first take your blood pressure and then write you out a prescription. This very same person happened to own the pharmacy across the road, so it was an easy hop, skip, and a jump to get your prescription filled. This man's lucrative business practices were lining his pockets on both sides of the silver dollar.

A veterinarian's assistant from the University of Wisconsin trained with Rocky at the gym and was willing to supply him with the injection steroids and administer them as well. Stages or cycles were still recommended in 1982 as they were eleven years before: eight weeks on the drugs and four weeks of off-time. For the eight week period, two to three shots per week were given, and ten pills a day were dropped. During the four-week layoff, nothing was administered or taken. Rocky followed instructions, went about his business, and waited on results. Practically overnight Rocky's powerful muscles seemed to magically blossom. In a three-month timeframe his bodyweight increased to 250 pounds.

The abusive steroid treatment on his physical body was the man's secret between himself and a couple of true friends at the gym. Sapphire would have never understood her husband's need for them because of her resentment toward every aspect of Rocky's obsession with weight training. Also, black market steroids were very expensive. The only way that he could afford to pay for the detrimental drugs was to accelerate his expense accounts. Exaggerating his expenses was only going to be temporary, in his mind. He could already visualize winning the Mr. America Over 40 title, with the endorsement offers and cash rolling in by the bushel.

Sapphire had a rather difficult time trying to understand her husband's strict daily eating requirements. Anabolic steroids were considered an appetite stimulant, and putting on weight was the key to building muscle mass. Rocky would consume a large dosage of calories every day until eight weeks before a competition. Then he would back off his calorie intake to almost nothing, carefully consuming a fat-free diet for the last two months.

Rocky had the labels on tuna fish cans memorized. He would only eat tuna canned in water, broiled fish, chicken without the Colonel's secret recipe, and broiled egg whites without the yolk. Dairy products, bread, pasta, sugar, sodium, and shredded wheat were all eliminated from his diet. In this man's mind, if he deviated from these strict rations, it would be like swallowing cyanide. All of Rocky's difficult long hours of hard work and dreams of winning would decease with that one fatal indulgence. His goal was to achieve 5% body fat, and by nibbling on a cold slice of pizza and popcorn late at night, would not account for this anorexic body-weight consumption. Rocky was more than willing to make this small eating sacrifice.

"Our grocery bill is outrageous, Norman," Sapphire would scream while watching her husband devour two broiled chickens at one sitting. "How about trying different pasta recipes or something that's a bit cheaper?" She knew what Norman's answer would be but still didn't want to give up on the idea of stretching their depleting food budget a little further.

"I can't have crap like that, Sapphire," Rocky would shout back. "I'm sure you know that, so just get off my ass." This bickering would sometimes turn into a screaming match.

Rocky would consume a large glass of orange juice before a workout, which would give him the sugar needed for an energy boost. He would guzzle gallons of a cola beverage that was caffeine-free and low in sodium.

The giant body builder had to settle for runner-up in the 1982 Mr. America Over 40 contest. That did not stop him from driving himself harder to win in 1983. Rocky increased his weight training time and also his steroid intake. He doubled his oral consumption to twenty pills a day and his injections to four or five times a week. The monetary expenses and potential health risks were adding up extremely fast, but he just had to win this time—even if it would cost him his life.

Rocky's amplified drug consumption sometimes turned into steroid rages at home, which were usually directed at his wife Sapphire. He could control his temper around customers and friends but had to vent off his frustrations around her. Did he really aim to hurt the one he loved? Or did Rocky really love Sapphire? Maybe he thought of her (as he did of his previous two wives) as a bothersome, nagging creature who plainly tried to stand in the way of his vivid dreams and obsessions. Rocky was simply a miserable excuse for an understanding and loving husband. A day in the life of the Rauch family was becoming unbearable for the deteriorating couple.

With Rocky's accelerated steroid abuse, a means of finding an alternative method to pay for this drug habit became increasingly difficult. At a buck and a half ($150) for a ten-vile box of Primobolan that lasted only two weeks, there was hardly a dime left over to pay for the orals that he was popping faster than kernels in an aluminum foil bag on a stove burner.

After saying a few prayers along the way, Rocky finally received the chance to make some money through his bodybuilding career.

While competing in Chicago, Jim Lenderson, the president of HealthRight International, approached Rocky after a photograph session. With his body fat a hair over 5% and his veins popping through his taut skin, Rocky looked very impressive to the president of the vitamin company. Jim asked him to endorse his company's products by featuring his photos in their upcoming sales campaign. "I'm at liberty to offer you the position of being a wholesale dealer for my company," explained Jim. "In this manner you may purchase our vitamins at dealer cost and in turn sell them to all your weight-lifting buddies to make extra cash money on the side."

Being the natural-born salesman that he was, Rocky jumped at this gracious opportunity to make some easy money selling vitamins. So when brand new rookies entered the gym where Rocky worked out and asked, "How did you get so huge, Rocky?" he would turn around and answer, "I take HealthRight International vitamin packages developed for morning and evening consumption, and I also drink their protein powder called Size." Naturally, the gullible new weightlifters would line up in droves to purchase every vitamin pack and can of protein powder they could possibly afford. Then they would come back for more after their supplies diminished. Rocky was raking in an easy $400 or $500 extra a month to pay for his steroid habit.

His conscience did slightly bother him as Rocky would tell these newcomers, "If you guys stay on these vitamins, in about seven or eight months you'll all be monsters." He felt like a hypocrite because to become that monster like he was advertising, he knew in his mind that it would take years of dedicated weightlifting and massive doses of steroids. But because of his financial situation, he had to conceal his feelings and milk the vitamin gravy train for all it was worth.

At forty-one years of age in 1983, Rocky felt better than ever with a driving force to train harder to win. He allowed absolutely nothing to stand in his way of reaching his goal of conquering the Mr. America Over 40 competition. Most other old-timers were out playing a weekend round of golf or maybe a tennis doubles match with their wives. Rocky was now cross-training between power lifting and bodybuilding, focusing all of his attention on the upcoming Wisconsin State Power Lifting Championship, the sport that physicians had told him to give up.

At the state championship, Rocky excelled by setting three new records in his weight class of 275 pounds. He bench pressed 420 pounds, squatted a masterful 650 pounds, and dead lifted 605. He felt a sense of pride and arrogance throughout his entire massive body when he mastered this contest with no noticeable side effects or pain from an old power lifting injury. The only pain that Rocky acquired was from the self-inflicting punishment on his body from pumping iron over a quarter-ton in weight.

The 1983 Mr. Wisconsin Over 35 competition had arrived when Sapphire announced that she had entirely enough of her husband's obsession. The couple had checked into a Milwaukee motel the day before the huge event, bringing Rocky's good friend Ray along for the ride. The threesome was just about ready to walk out the door for dinner when Sapphire hit Rocky with a surprise: "I'm real tired of all this bodybuilding crap, Norman. If you compete in this stupid tournament tomorrow, I will file for a divorce and leave you for good."

"You have got to be kidding me, Sapphire!" exclaimed Norman. His eyes turned as cold as steel when his wife's ultimatum began to seep into his mind. "I've been working my fucking ass off to get ready for this competition, and you're telling me the night before that you'll leave me if I compete? What kind of shit is this, anyway?"

Sapphire's tone of voice became hatefully defiant. "That's right, fathead. I will definitely divorce you. You need to decide by tomorrow if it's going to be competing with barbells all the time or being with me."

Ray sat on an awkward coffee table like a bump on a log, wishing he could disappear. He anticipated a gruesome showdown to the finale with only one winner. The question was what would that winner win? Would Sapphire win her way out of a depleting marriage? Would Rocky be a king in the weightlifting world minus another wife?

Rocky was too disgusted to go to battle with a woman at that moment. Instead, he glared piercing icicle daggers into Sapphire's side of the battle zone. "Well, if that is how you feel about this matter, then you had better pack your bags and find yourself a way home." Without giving his wife a chance to rehash his last statement over in her mind, Norman snatched his coat, swung the front door open, shoved Ray through it, and left.

The next day at the big event, without Sapphire in the crowd to cheer him on, Rocky won the state championship with honors. His wife's threat phased out to be mostly talk and very little action. She did not leave her Rocky. But still upset with her husband's true love, Sapphire kept the hatred of his sport inside her and refused to fly to Los Angeles with him when Rocky competed for the big Mr. America Over 40 title the following August.

During his airline flight to one of the largest cities in the States, Rocky utilized this spacious serenity to contemplate his future as a bodybuilder. He was all alone, trying to create a vivid photograph of himself being displayed in all of the top-shelf fitness and bodybuilding magazines. Rocky could picture his telephone ringing off of the wall, as companies from all over would want him to advertise their products. He really wanted his wife to love his sport just maybe a fraction of as much as he did and to prove to her that hard work and dedication had paid off. He still had hopes of her coming around and taking an interest in his hobby—or possibly a lifetime dream career that would have him rolling in the dough. All Rocky had to do for his hopes and dreams to come true was to win.

Of course, that's much easier said than done.

Rocky's super-ego took him wandering even deeper into the future. "Winning this Mr. America Over 40 championship will only be the beginning for me. I will not stop there by any means. My ultimate goal is to be the first man over 40 to win the regular Mr. America contest in 1984. I'm sure that I will be competing against young guys in their twenties and thirties, but what the hell! My vascular body is every bit as dynamic as these young punks' bodies are, and I have facial expressions and body language that offer character, experience, and just plain natural instincts. I have rolled with the punches ever since one of those punks cracked my jawbone in two places. The judges out there would surely choose maturity over a wet behind the ears, peach-fuzzed, baby-faced kid, wouldn't they?

"I see no reason why I can't claim victory after the Mr. America contest in 1984, do you, Lord? But first things first, I need to focus my attention on winning this next Over 40 contest. So I pray to you, my dear Lord, can you please help me out this time? I've been trying to be a good child of yours, but it's not easy. The world out there is very difficult to live in, let alone be master of. I beg of you to help let the judges recognize my ability to perform in the upcoming competition. I am very sorry for my sins. Amen."

A health club in Racine, Wisconsin, had sponsored Rocky in this Over 40 championship. Compliments of the health club, he had the privacy of a condominium in Santa Monica on the beach for one week, airfare completely paid for, and promised future endorsements if he dominated this contest. How could Rocky not win? He was ripped and more than ready for action. Rocky's bodyweight was a perfect 219 pounds and his body fat a mere 5%

because of the extra bicycling and running he had tacked onto his schedule in the past two months. This man of superhuman strength had trained harder for this competition than any other contest in his entire life.

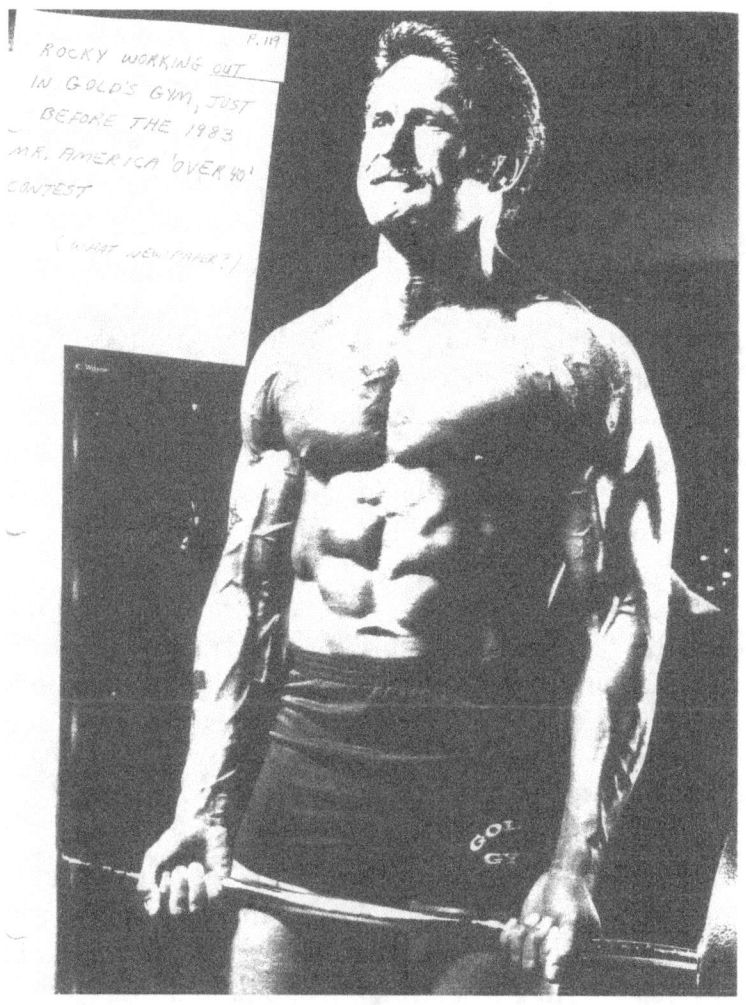

ROCKY WORKING OUT
IN GOLD'S GYM, JUST
BEFORE THE 1983
MR. AMERICA 'OVER 40'
CONTEST

(WHAT NEWSPAPER?)

Arriving in California one week before the competition, Rocky still trained in the mornings at Gold's Gym, lay out in the hot sand to acquire that all important bronze tan, and practiced posing in front of a full-length mirror at the condo in the evenings. A few days before the big event, Tom Platts, a former Mr. Universe, approached Rocky at the gym and stated, "You look like you might be retaining water, Mr. Rauch."

"I don't see how," answered Rocky. "I've really been watching my diet."

"You've got a stove where you're staying, right?" asked Tom. "You should be eating broiled fish, and that's it. No egg whites, no chicken, no tuna. Just three ounces of broiled fish every six hours, around the clock. Tonight set your alarm clock before bed, and then wake up and broil three ounces of fish. Trust me on this."

"Really?" asked Rocky.

"Really," stated Tom. "Every six hours your body needs fish. Then the day before the competition, I want you to quit with the fish and start trickle carbing. Carbohydrates will make your muscles swell. Approximately every three hours, alternate between eating one-fourth of an apple and half of a plain white baked potato."

Rocky sincerely thanked the former Mr. Universe for his expertise and then stopped by the local market and stocked up on a handful of red delicious apples, a few large white sprouting potatoes, and a couple of pounds of fish. He faithfully followed the advice of the former competitor for the remaining three days. When all ordinary people were sleeping, Rocky would be up in the middle of the night preparing his tasteless skimpy portions, as Tom's schedule precisely mandated.

Thursday afternoon, Rocky stretched out his towel in the sand, lubed up his body with sunscreen, lay back and fell asleep. When he woke up from his nap an hour later, he found himself surrounded by a couple of fellows. "I hope that this is still part of my dream," Rocky thought. Was this another gay rights movement? Gay men were starting to swarm in like pollen-hungry killer bees!

"May I please rub some more suntan oil on your delicious body, Mr. Muscleman?" asked one of the happy-go-lucky guys, licking his lips.

"Can I take you out to lunch, my big strong man?" asked another in his best feminine voice.

Rocky prided himself on being a dedicated American heterosexual and was very offended by this disturbing crowd of nonconformists. He flew off the handle, growling out a few curse words, and then he grabbed his towel and supplies and headed for a more secluded spot on the beach. As he ventured farther up the beach through the burning sand, he also had no clue that he was being trailed by a secret admiring private eye. After the muscleman situated himself on his towel scented with sweat, this gay fellow approached him.

"I'm very sorry about my friends, mister," apologized the gay guy. "They can be a bit outspoken when they line their eyes on a big man like you."

"Well, okay, but I'm straight, Bruce," quoted Rocky. "So just leave me alone and go back to your own kind."

"I understand," answered the guy, "but I'm a professional photographer. See?" He held up his leather camera case to prove his statement.

"Yeah, so what?" asked Rocky.

"So I would love to photograph you, if you wouldn't mind, sir," said the cameraman.

Rocky's large ego clicked in as his mind did an about-face. "A new set of prints might be just what the doctor ordered," thought Rocky. "How much would you charge me?"

"Not a mere dime, sir," stated the photographer. "It would be an honor and a privilege. I've never seen a body as fantastic as yours before."

"Let's not get fresh here, buddy," snickered Rocky. "And please don't try to hit on me like your gay partners did, all right?"

"You have yourself a deal," said the photographer. "And I will have as many copies made for you as you want of your best poses, Mr....what do I call you?"

"You may call me the Real Rocky," answered Rocky.

"That name does fit your style, I must say," said the photographer.

Knowing that he was in superior physical shape, this photographer's offer was too enticing to refuse. Some of these professional snapshot artists were outright expensive, and with his budget always straining to keep up with the exorbitant cost of steroids, Rocky could see no reason not to allow this professional to photograph him to his heart's content. So the massive muscular man stood up with the horizon at his backside and gave the camera guy something to shoot. The final results were simply magnificent. The honest photographer kept his word and sent Rocky numerous copies of the best poses on the roll.

The day of the competition had finally arrived. There was an afternoon and an evening show. Norman Rauch was competing with twenty-six other contestants and was elated with the good fortune of drawing the twenty-seventh position. This meant that he would be the last and final bodybuilder to impress the judges, with the images of the first assembly line posers beginning to fade away from their memory. Anxious and ready to go into the limelight, Rocky was trying to calm his mind while flexing his tight muscles in the full-length mirrored warm-up room.

Then, without any previous warning signals, a near disaster occurred. He could feel his calves and quadriceps lock up on him like the high security prison cell gates at Statesville. The pain was so unbearable that Rocky could hardly walk as his muscles were cramping. Bent over and almost on his knees crying for help, he could not hold back his tear ducts from overflowing. His pain became more excruciating by the minute, and his mental anguish was so severe that the only thing that Rocky could think about was, "Why me, Lord? Please don't let this happen again." He was finished, locked up. He would have to withdraw from the competition.

The expeditor just happened to witness the big man in distress and rushed over to his side. "Here. Eat these," the man said while reaching out to hand Rocky a bag of potato chips.

"I can't eat chips," Rocky said exasperatedly. "I will bloat up like a blubber whale from the fat and sodium."

"No, you won't, sir—not until tomorrow, anyway," answered the expeditor. "What your body needs this very moment is salt. Trust me. I've seen this happen before. Hurry up and eat a handful, and your body will uncramp."

Without another option to think about at the moment and just minutes before his name would be called, Rocky had no other available choice. So he followed the man's instructions by consuming the chips in rapid succession and then waiting for about two minutes. The minutes seemed like hours. Then, all of a sudden, something miraculous happened. The severe pain subsided, his muscles unclenched, and Rocky was able to stand up straight again. "Thank you very much, sir," Norman said graciously, "and thank you, Lord in heaven!"

"Not a problem," said the advisor. "Glad to have been of service."

When he heard his name mentioned over the public address system, Rocky strutted gracefully over to his starting position on stage. Rocky turned on the charm with the perfect pearly white smile and performed his natural and mandatory poses like he had been doing this since childbirth. Finally it was all over, and his huge body and ego were in a state of exuberance. But he still could not be sure that he had won the championship until the judges had their scorecards calculated.

Rocky eventually learned about his victory from the same person who helped him through his time of need. "You won!" exclaimed the expeditor.

"I owe you big time," Rocky said gratefully before returning to the stage in front of his admiring fans.

The preliminary round of the heavyweight division championship was a first place rap for Rocky that he had snug tight in his hip back pocket by now. This glowing champion headed straight back for the beach, on the other side this time, to bask in the rays of God's sunshine. If he did as well as he had during the daylight hours, Rocky would become the 1983 Mr. America Over 40 champion before both hands on the theatrical arena grandfather clock struck midnight.

A total of five finalists were competing that evening for the gold. In the preliminaries of the daytime contest, one winner was declared in each weight category from bottom to top: lightweight, middle weight, light heavyweight, and super heavyweight. Rocky had been judged to be the finest in his division, the heavyweight category. All five of these contestants would be competing for the Mr. America title. Rocky felt the rush of his life knowing that he would walk away with the prestigious title.

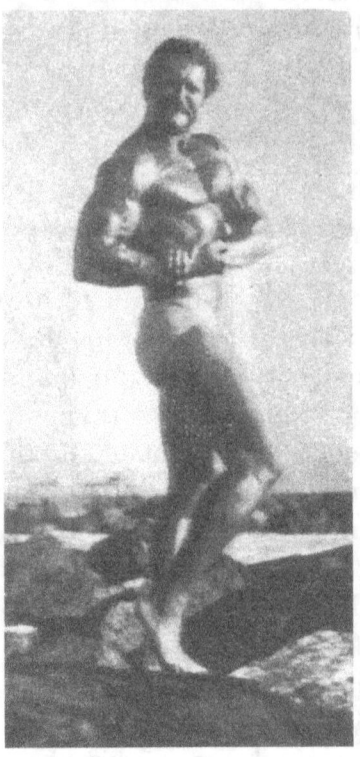

It was no longer a dream on the beach; this was the real thing. "We present to you our heavyweight champion, Mr. Norman Rauch," came the voice over the loudspeaker system. Rocky took a couple of deep breaths, walked up on stage, and went into action. He did his natural poses first, then the mandatory still-life shots for the cameras, and finally the sensational sensual part of his act, the one-minute pose-down that was set to seductive music. The sounds added heightened drama as the graceful muscular man maneuvered every part of his body from one striking stance to another. In a rather slow, deliberate fashion, Rocky kicked in some gentle ballet-like movements. When his allotment of time was through, the cheers from the audience were deafening. Based on the crowd appreciation, there was no doubt that if those thousands of spectators were judges, Rocky would have been declared the winner on the spot. But the audience's opinion was not the deciding factor; seven sophisticated judges would make the final decision on who would take home the national title. Rocky could only stand in the wings and hope that those judges would side with the screaming fans.

After the judges had a brief tabulation period, the winning announcement was made. "Our big winner tonight—and we mean huge—is from the dairyland state of Wisconsin. Will Mr. Norman 'Rocky' Rauch please come up to center stage to be crowned the 1983 Mr. America Over 40 King?" The audience went nuts as the ultimate high struck the big man's ego. Rocky's first instinct was to pinch himself to make sure he wasn't still dreaming on the beach. He was presented with handshakes and a dynamite trophy after he strutted back up on that stage for one last title-winning pose. It was a lifelong dream come true. This massive bodybuilder would always remember that evening in Hemmings Auditorium as the most exciting night of his career.

Even though Sapphire had point-blank refused to accompany her husband to Los Angeles and was totally non-supportive through this whole competition, Rocky still felt compelled to phone her and seek her approval. Surely she would be ecstatic for him as this night went into the history books. Or would she even care?

He dialed the telephone number and waited impatiently for his wife to pick up. "Hello, Sapphire. It's me, Rocky. I won, baby. I won the title!"

The female tone on the other end was cold and slurred. "You did not wi…win. Don't lie to me. I need the truth."

"I am not lying, honey. I scored a victory tonight in this huge competition. I won it all!" yelled Rocky.

Sapphire shouted back, "And I suppose you'll be coming home tom…tomorrow and expect your lovely wife to pick you up at the airport."

"That would be nice," said Rocky in a tone of voice that descended from a spectacular high to a disenchanted low.

"Well, I won't be there for you," answered Rocky's wife. "I'm going up north for a couple of days."

Rocky questioned her, "Where are you going up north?"

"Just out and about with friends of mine," stated Sapphire, "so I'm sor...sorry, but you'd better make different travel plans from the airport."

Based on her snide remarks and her tongue whiplashes, Rocky was definitely surprised that his wife did not slam the phone down to make his ears ring. Immature or not, the outraged husband felt that he deserved that last word. With snake-like venom injected into his vocal chords, Rocky yelled "Get ripped!" and threw the telephone across the room.

Despite feeling a bit lonely and let down from the conversation with his wife, Rocky still had that arrogant attitude directly within his grasp. While packing for the flight home, he laid out his best pair of tight, seductive shorts and a tank top to impress the stews and the peanut gallery fan club for his adventure forward. He wanted someone to make a big deal out of this victory that was the ultimate goal of his life. He finally was a star!

But Jesus spoke at that very moment into Rocky's memory, "My son, you must take pride in your accomplishments, but never forget the true souls that have led you on your journey forth to venture onto the pathway of the forgiveness of your sins and to your eternal destination."

Rocky was overwhelmed for a few minutes by his thoughts from his Creator, but then somehow thinking of his wardrobe stuck into his brain. Was it the advice of the red devil himself? With his massive muscles bulging, there was no way that Rocky could simply dissolve into the United Airlines upholstery. The muscular monument would be as conspicuous in his tank top as Superman would have been in his red cape.

On the flight home a stewardess took one look at this hunk of a man and just had to ask, "Who are you, Mr. America or somebody?"

Rocky was already for his opening reply, "As a matter of fact, doll face, I am." He told the story of winning this spectacular competition, and the word quickly spread like the Santa Ana winds. The flight attendants inflated his ego even farther with verbal compliments and special attention. The party was on. They fueled him with complimentary champagne and made extra time to stop by his aisle seat and gush all over this magnificent-looking creature. Remaining exactly where he wanted to be, in the spotlight on this flight, was exactly what Rocky needed after the conversation with his wife. He loved every minute of attention and recognition.

After the plane made its descent and landing, the glorious super hero spotted his friend Ray and his daughter Jennifer waiting impatiently for his arrival inside the terminal at O'Hare in Chicago. Jennifer was now a teenager and was very proud of her father and thrilled to death for his victory. Ray was elated as well, sharing stories and throwing in compliments on the road back to Milwaukee. At four o'clock in the morning the three of them entered an empty house with the telephone ringing off the wall in the darkness. Rocky thought for a moment that it might be Sapphire calling with second thoughts, regretting not picking him up at the airport and wanting to apologize. His hurt feelings were still not ready to accept her apology just yet.

But it was not Sapphire. It was Rocky's mother Dorothy calling with some startling news, "I'm so glad that you answered the phone, Norman. It's your father. Henry had a severe heart attack. They rushed him off to the Fort Wayne Hospital tonight."

"I'm on my way there, Mother," spoke her son, getting his second wind from hearing that painful news. He did not even know how to get a hold of his wife by phone because he didn't know where the hell she was. Instead, his daughter went along to visit her grandfather at his bedside. It would be the last time that either of them would see Henry alive.

As they entered the hospital room, Rocky was the first person to speak. "How are you feeling this morning, Dad?" Tears filled his eyes as the big man pulled his chair closer to his frail-looking father.

"Not too bad, son," Henry managed to get out in a weaker-than-usual tone of voice. A faint smile arose from his parched lips. "Did you win?"

Rocky latched on tight to his father's hand with fear that Henry might see the light at any moment and leave this earth with God's guardian angels from above. "I did, Dad. I won."

"That's wonderful, son. I'm very proud of you," whispered Henry.

Rocky's brother Charlie was also in the hospital wing, but he was not so proud of his brother as his father was, even though he claimed to be. Rocky felt a sense of jealousy simmering below the surface of his younger brother's respectful congratulations. Although his younger brother Charlie was just as accomplished in his world—especially academically, with an electrical engineering degree from Indiana Tristate College—it was fairly obvious that he resented his older brother's latest achievement.

Charlie was also the vice president of cellular pager division for Motorola. His father actually was the one who forced Charlie to go to college to become an engineer; Charlie wanted to be a welder. In their younger days and still somewhat to that day Charlie felt that he always had to compete with his brother because Rocky was so often in the limelight. Rocky had been able to develop a closer relationship with Henry later on in life but had not been able to bond with his only brother.

Henry died three months later, and at first a huge burden was placed on Rocky's mind because father and son had become quite good friends toward Henry's final years. Rocky's main regret was that his father's premature death robbed them of spending more time together.

By no means did Sapphire want to attend Henry's funeral with her husband, but with Rocky's persistence, she put her hostilities toward him aside for one day and accompanied him to Allentown. Even to an intelligent spider living on their bedroom walls, it would have been obvious that the couple's marriage was over, but Rocky and Sapphire remained husband and wife for several more years.

CHAPTER 8
THE APPLE OF HIS MOST
SEDUCTIVE THOUGHTS

The brand new Mr. America Over 40 did not receive the national endorsements that he had planned on, although he was being paid as much as $500 to make local appearances in the Wisconsin area. Rocky's ego was reaching for the stars when he and Sapphire moved into their new home in Pewaukee. He was pretty certain that these fine citizens would want to know the celebrity status of their new neighbor. After all, the big-time Deforest newspaper had written an exclusive story about his glorious win in California, so this he could only assume that his hometown newspaper would want to as well. Rocky visited the local paper one day on foot and offered, "I just thought maybe you guys would like to know that my wife and I just moved into town. How would you like to run a front-page story on me?"

With local news being somewhat scarce in this tiny village, the newspaper's editor seemed very pleased to write a feature story. "I'll send a reporter out to your house on Saturday. We welcome you with open arms to our community." He greeted Rocky with an extended handshake instead of a bear hug.

Many years later, Rocky could only chuckle and feel somewhat embarrassed about how his inexcusable vanity was back then. "I can't believe that I actually did that. It must have been that devil in disguise that gave me so much confidence to go out and ask a newspaper to cover my story as some kind of a big shot. My Lord had carried me this far with only one set of footprints in the sand. I should have realized then, that pursuing my excessive conceited dreams would not make me a superstar at the gateway to heaven's harvest."

The newspaper sent a female reporter out to their new house on Saturday. Sapphire was steamed about the whole ordeal. She was very tired of her husband being in the spotlight all the time and treating her like an old maid. "Well, here is what old maids do," she thought. Sapphire didn't get rambunctious at that very moment. She continued cleaning house in her old blue jeans and tattered sweatshirt when the professional-looking reporter showed up in her color-coordinated business outfit. Rocky invited the reporter into his living room and asked her to have a seat on the comfortable recliner. The outspoken reporter started to ask many favorable questions in Rocky's direction while Sapphire kept fidgeting and waving cleaning apparatuses at her.

Slightly irritated with this situation, the reporter asked, "How do you feel about your husband winning the Mr. America Over 40 contest, Mrs. Rauch? You must be very proud of him." Rocky covered his face and shook his head dramatically in despair as he remembered the lonesome feeling.

Sapphire stopped dead in her track and screeched, "I want you to take this down word for word so you can quote me accurately for all your readers to acknowledge." The reporter sat up a little bit straighter in the recliner with her ink pen ready to spear at her notepad at an instant's notice. "I think this all sucks, big time!"

Rocky was very embarrassed at that moment, and so was the reporter. She could not believe what she had just heard. After another series of questions directed at Mr. Rauch, the reporter said that she had all the necessary information for her story and made a final excuse to get out of there. The article was written without any input from Rocky's miserable wife's perspective. Sapphire was still slamming down Rhine wine like there was no tomorrow. She had probably doubled her intake that day because of her husband's obsession with being such a macho man.

Rocky could find no way to get through to her to heal this wounded marriage. His wife's resentment of him had festered into an untreatable open abrasion by then. Although Sapphire still had the ability to function in her occupation at the Milwaukee Blood Center, evening and weekend moods alternated between blurred sauce dazes and raging fits. Things were getting so nasty between them that Rocky found himself living in motels whenever his job would let him. His career as a traveling salesman afforded him that escape.

One Thursday afternoon while in Burlington on business, a customer of Rocky's proposed a deal that the big guy could not refuse. Mark said, "I know about your situation at home, and I think maybe you should stay here with me tonight and have a little fun. There's a big street dance tonight, and I believe you'll enjoy yourself. I'll make a couple of quick phone calls and get you a blind date with a real fox! How does that sound?"

"Make the call, buster. I'm hanging out," announced Rocky. "Just give me a few minutes to put on something more revealing for my blind date." Rocky dressed in his customary summer's evening attire, a tank top and shorts with GOLD'S GYM printed on the bottom left side. Granted, he felt cooler in his skimpy clothing, but he usually underdressed to impress the sexy ladies and to intimidate the men with his incredible Hulk-like physique.

The two gentlemen took off to the street dance like teenagers with raging hormones, thinking that they both might get lucky on this Thursday afternoon. Rocky's blind date could not meet him until later, so the first stop on the agenda was the beer tent. The cobblestone streets were crowded with numerous people, with the aroma of delicious chocolate assaulting their taste buds from the nearby candy factory. Beer for the gents and chocolate for the gals. What more could anyone ask for?

"There's a real live fox," shouted Rocky, looking in Mark's direction.

"Where at?" asked Mark.

"Over there," answered Rocky. "See that blonde over there in tight jeans wearing a cowboy hat ?" As he drank from his plastic cup, Rocky savored the cold beer while savoring the vision of the gorgeous cowgirl in the distance. "Man, would I ever like to meet that chick. Ride 'em, cowboy!"

Mark continued to play the role of Rocky's boastful pimp. "You want to meet her? Not a problem, my friend." Mark walked away, making his usual stride through the crowd toward the gal. Rocky could only assume that his buddy Mark had faded away to fetch the blonde girl he had requested, so he casually focused his attention elsewhere, trying not to be conspicuous. But when Mark didn't return with the dream girl, Rocky's eyes started to scan the distant horizon for them. His efforts were comfortably put to rest as neither one of the two were anywhere to be seen.

A short time later, Rocky was momentarily startled by the voice of a sweet, confident cowgirl. "I'm from the National Bun Society." He spun around in his seat and was delighted to see his dream girl make her introduction.

"She must have been handpicked in the Garden of Eden," thought Rocky.

"I'm doing photographs for our annual calendar," said the blonde gal with the cowgirl hat still in place. "We still have a couple of months left open. Which one would you like, big fellow?"

Rocky played along. "Well, my birthday just happens to come along every March, when that old lion tamer puts the brakes on the horrible wind chill elements. Then right after my birthday, old man winter will have been defeated and the shepherds will have a one dog night instead of three."

"You're pulling my leg, aren't you?" asked the delicious blonde. She went on to smile seductively and say, "I think that I still have March open."

Rocky snickered, "Well, since this is a bun calendar, I just need to know one thing. I have to know if you'd like my picture with or without."

"With or without what?" she asked. "Oh, you mean fresh and undressed, popping straight out of the oven." The cowgirl's grin remained coy as her cheeks reddened enough to suggest that she was slightly embarrassed by her forwardness.

Rocky caught on and shyly smiled back. "I guess we need to discuss that. Can I buy you a beer?"

The two were enjoying each other's company until Rocky remembered his blind date. "I'd like to spend more time with you, Trudy, but my friend Mark arranged a date for me this evening. I should go meet her now."

"Really?" asked Trudy. "Well, I guess that's too bad, Norman. I'd like to get to know you better. So maybe I'll see you later?" Her devilish eyes haunted Rocky from beneath the shadow of her cowgirl hat, and when she smiled at him, he found himself lost in her magical disposition. He felt drawn to her, as if by some unexplainable magnetic force. Rocky knew that he had to see this goddess once again and could not wait for what the future had in store.

"Listen, I don't even know this blind date," Rocky said, feeling a bit disturbed. "I want more than anything to be with you tonight, but I said that I would meet her, and I really wouldn't feel right not showing up. I'll just tell her that I'm sick or something, and then I could meet you at the corner bar at eleven o'clock."

"All right," said Trudy. "I'll be at the Corner Bar waiting for you at eleven."

Rocky had no qualms about blowing off his date, especially when he found out that she had red hair. He had never really hit it off with a redhead before and did not want to try to figure out the fired up mood swings of this one. After a couple of minutes of dialogue, it came to Rocky's attention that his date lived on a pig farm with her parents. His mind started to make comparisons as his blind date was speaking, and the pig-farming redhead was no match for a blonde cowgirl in tight Wranglers.

"Listen, I'm feeling a bit under the weather right now," spoke Rocky as he cuffed his neck with his right forefinger and thumb and let out a fake cough.

"Oh my goodness," said the redhead. "I hope you're going to be all right."

"Yeah, I think maybe it's the flu," answered Rocky. "I have a headache and am starting to feel achy all over. Maybe we should have this date another night."

"I'm sorry that you are not feeling well," spoke the girl, "and I hate to bother you about this, but I need a ride home. I don't have a car."

"Sure. No problem," said Rocky, "I can take you back to your pig farm. Where exactly is it?"

"It's kind of out of town a ways in the country," replied his date.

Rocky was happy to oblige…anything to get her out of the picture so he could rejoin the apple of his eye. As he kept to himself and looked at his wristwatch every five minutes or so, he started to think that maybe this farm was in Illinois rather than Wisconsin. But he did some calculations in his head and figured that he could still get rid of his date and meet up with Trudy at eleven o'clock as planned.

With a touch of sweat on his brow, he made it back to the bar on the corner where he thought that he was to meet Trudy with not one minute to spare. Rocky picked a table for two without a crowded view of the main entrance, ordered a brew, and waited. Every time that he ordered another beer, he checked his watch. After the third one at 11:45, Rocky was wondering where she could possibly be. When the waitress approached her customer as both hands on the clock struck midnight, Rocky abruptly stood up and replied, "No more for me, thank you. I'm out of here." His mind went into a head-spin as he walked out of the bar and grill. He had been stood up by a girl he barely knew, whom he had completely misjudged. During the short time that they were together, she had seemed so genuine, down to earth, and honest.

Out in the street, there were different cliques of people, each having fun in their own way. Rocky was like a foreigner in this town of Burlington as he looked around, trying to get his bearings on where he was at. He looked above the crowd and spotted a sign that read: THE CORNER BAR. "Boy am I ever a dumbass," Rocky thought. He could not believe his own eyes. There was actually a bar in this crazy town called The Corner Bar. As he opened the front door, Norm could only hope that Trudy was inside still waiting on him to make an appearance.

The Corner Bar was rocking and rolling with a party-time atmosphere. Within a few seconds, Rocky found Trudy sandwiched between two men. As Rocky passed by her to get to an empty table, the cute blonde was laughing and carrying on like there was no tomorrow. When they were close enough to be face to face, the cowgirl offered Rocky a casual acknowledgement, "Hi!"

Feeling like just another piece of meat being discarded, Rocky grumbled back the same word with less feeling and kept on walking to one of the back tables to be alone. He had expected the blonde babe to fall all over him, out of reach of the two hungry masculine sharks that were surrounding her. A sense of depression hit Rocky like a ton of bricks as his mind wandered back to his home life. He was tired of drinking alone and feeling the blues.

A while later, Trudy pranced over to Rocky's table and said, "I see that you made it."

"Yeah, I went to the bar on the corner across the street and waited there for you for an hour," explained Rocky, feeling a bit guilty and uneasy.

"I'm sorry about that," answered Trudy, "but I thought that you knew your way around this town. Would you like to dance with me?"

It was plain and simple to see from Rocky's point of view that this gorgeous creature was more interested in being a party animal than spending some time alone with him. He had felt that they had a chemistry going on between them and was rather offended that she had not felt this as well. Her frivolous body language toward him only fueled his feelings of rejection more now than ever. "I don't dance."

After that overwhelming response to her politeness, the blonde cowgirl felt rejected also. But she was still having a merry old time and was not going to let the remark of this muscle-head ruin her mood. "All right, be that way," she stated and pranced back over by the bar like a glowing reindeer to rejoin her two companions.

Rocky was hoping that he could just pick up his bags and leave to catch the next boxcar ride to nowhere, but instead he ordered one more beer for good measure. He had this deep fascination with her, something that he really couldn't explain at the moment. While sipping on the last few ounces, Rocky found himself focusing on a vision of an undressed blonde-haired goddess, appearing on a white stallion with silver reins and bit, who would take him away from all this. Then reality struck back, and Rocky's huge neck was getting stiff from exchanging secretive glances with the cowgirl of his dreams. He would stare at her when he thought she wasn't looking his way and vice-versa. And what the lonely hunk of a man thought he saw was a showgirl just having a ball with her male buddies, dancing, laughing, and singing along with the band. The more fun it looked like Trudy was having, the more steamed Rocky became.

Finally, one of the guys that she was with broke the ice and approached the muscleman. "Hello, I'm Harley."

"Like in Davidson," Rocky smirked.

"I wish," he said, "but seriously, Trudy really wants to get to know you."

"Really? You're serious?" asked Rocky. "Well, she certainly isn't acting like it."

"I think there's been a misunderstanding," replied Harley. "I haven't seen Trudy in years. We used to be friends in high school. We just sort of bumped into each other tonight and are trying to catch up." Harley sat down next to Rocky, trying to be as reasonable and friendly as possible. "Oh, and that other guy? He's the son of the dentist that Trudy used to work for. He's also an obnoxious son-of-a-bitch. He keeps hitting on her, but she's not interested in him at all. It's you that she wants."

Rocky smirked and spoke, "You really think so?"

"Yeah. I think she'd be very grateful if you would toss him out the back door and steal her heart," snickered Harley. "Just don't tell her that I encouraged you to do that." Harley stood back up to go back and join his friends after being forced to play matchmaker. When Rocky didn't comment one way or another, Harley walked back over by the bar wondering how his old high school chum could be so interested in a giant who seemed so cold and distant.

For about another half an hour, Rocky drank alone pondering moodily, with tears dripping into his beer. To strangers, his frame of mind and body language made no sense. The big hunk of a man was self-centered, somewhat spoiled, and accustomed to feeling superior because of women falling all over him. This blonde knockout was not gushing over him. In fact, Trudy made him feel like he was invisible, which was very hard to handle after being in the limelight so many times.

It was getting late, and the bar lights started to flicker, giving that ungrateful warning signal that it was time for last call. Rocky knew in the back of his mind that he had to make his decision right now, or not at all. Ready or not, he would have to overpower his humiliation and make his move or walk straight out the door and never return. On the spur of the moment, Rocky walked passed Trudy, then slowed down and turned his head, "Would you like to go out for coffee?"

"Where to?" she asked, cautiously trying to protect her own deep emotions.

"You can choose the place," Rocky replied, "I believe that I already proved I'm not very familiar with this town."

"Where are you staying tonight?" Trudy asked.

"I don't have a spot to hang my hat yet," answered Rocky. He had checked out of his motel that morning with the intentions of going back to Pewaukee until Mark had invited him to stay.

"I live in Lake Geneva," Trudy spoke. "You can follow me into town if you would like."

Following behind her car, weaving on the Wisconsin hills, Rocky felt that her driving skills were disoriented from too much alcohol.

Upon arriving safely, the cowgirl led the way into her mobile home living room and defensively said, "You may stay here tonight, on the couch or the beanbag. The choice is yours. But you will not be sleeping with me. Understand? Now with my ground rules established, I'll go make that coffee."

"Aye-aye, madam," Rocky chuckled. Even after coffee they were both pretty well wiped out to do anything other than sleep. Since the couch was a four-foot long loveseat and he wanted to stretch out rather than sleep in the fetal position, he chose the beanbag chair on the floor.

The next morning Rocky woke up to the smell of smoked Canadian bacon sizzling in a frying pan. His nostrils and taste buds told him to go directly into the kitchen, while his aching back, neck, and shoulders told him that he was too stiff to move. He actually had to do a reverse triceps pushup on a nearby existing chair to stand up and get motivated.

Trudy decided to wake up early to show her house guest some hospitality by cooking him a delicious breakfast. After sipping on his cooling coffee, Rocky felt recharged by the caffeine jolt, and his muscles started behaving themselves. He acquired the courage once again to ask her out. "Is there someplace that I can meet you for lunch?"

"There's a great place that I like to go to called Charlie-O's," answered Trudy with a gleam in her eye. Rocky was greatly aroused by her illustrious smile and mesmerized by her body language.

"Just give me the directions on how to get to this restaurant," replied Rocky, "and I'll meet you there for lunch. I can't wait to show you off." After making some sales calls from the mobile home, he had to shove off and run some errands. He couldn't stop thinking about the attraction he had for this five-foot-two, blonde, blue-eyed beauty. It was not only a sexual attraction but a deeper feeling of them being drawn together, almost as their first meeting had been fate. It was like two lost souls destined to be together, handpicked by the Lord himself before the beginning of time. At least for Rocky, it was truly love at first sight.

After getting to know each other a little better over lunch, Rocky knew that he had to see her again. "Listen, I've got to drive over to Rockford on business this afternoon," he explained. "Why don't I meet you here at six o'clock, and we'll have dinner. What do you say?"

Trudy felt at that moment the same magnetic attraction toward this man, possibly in the same manner that he felt about her. So she readily agreed to make his acquaintance once again at Charlie-O's restaurant. "I'll see you there, Norman. Please don't be late." She gave him a great big kiss on the lips.

As Trudy sat alone at the restaurant with the hands of the clock tick-tocking toward 7:30, she began to think that her date had played a deceitful trick on her. There could be no excuse for such tardiness an hour and a half after they were supposed to meet. She was coming to grips with the realization that she had been stood up. This little stunt that her man had pulled off filled her mind with huge disappointment and a sense of frustration and anger. How could Trudy have misjudged this jerk to hurt her pride so dearly? Her intention was to swallow the last gulp in her beverage glass and make a break for the back door. She didn't want to perceive the thought of all these customers talking about how she had been left alone to brood.

Then her peripheral vision caught sight of this large hunk of a man rushing through the doorway like he was late for his own funeral. Rocky was juggling a bouquet of flowers in one hand and a small, loudly-wrapped box in the other. He had a look of urgency on his face.

"I'm sorry I'm late," he explained, as he extended out his muscular arms with the gifts. "I bought these things for you."

"You're an hour and a half late because you stopped to buy me some gifts to make me feel better?" Trudy asked with a bit of sarcasm in her voice.

"No, I'm late because I got this phone call from L&M Construction here in Lake Geneva just before I was on my way to meet you," replied Rocky. "They needed a swimming pool panel that my boss had me deliver to them. It was just bad timing. That's all." As further proof, he pulled a business card out of his inside jacket pocket and showed it to her. "See? Have you ever heard of this construction company before?"

Disbelief was written all over Trudy's face. "Did you see a bald man there by the name of Mick Thompson?"

"Not that I can remember," stated Rocky. "Why do you ask?"

"Because that bald idiot that I'm talking about is my ex-husband," said Trudy.

"You must be kidding," snickered Rocky. "You're saying that shifty Mick Thompson is your ex-husband? I'm very surprised."

"Well, wasn't he there?" she asked once again to make sure.

"No. Lenny was there," answered Rocky, "and also Drake and Pike and their mother Lora." Then all of a sudden it hit Rocky that he did not even know Trudy's last name. "So you're Trudy Thompson?"

"Let me assure you in name only," said Trudy. "I have not one wafer of interest in that family or their construction business.

"Ahh, you brought me flowers, my big gorgeous man," said Trudy, starting to realize that Rocky just might be for real.

Rocky spent that night with his apple blossom as well as almost every night after that. He became quite masterful in lying to his legal wife Sapphire, always making up excuses as to why he couldn't be there. Rocky knew that his marriage to his wife was very much over, but he had a hard time dealing with that. If it would take until his dying days to be rid of the third gem in his life, so be it. Rocky so much wanted to be with the girl of his dreams forever and be able to call her his own, Mrs. Trudy Rauch.

Sapphire's father swung by Rocky's house one Friday night with his girlfriend for a drink. The four of them were all supposed to go to a fish fry together. Her father took Norm aside and said that he was very concerned about his daughter's drinking. Norm answered, "I'm also very upset with Sapphire's obsession with the bottle. She begins her morning at ten o'clock sharp with a large plastic cup of wine and doesn't stop indulging until she plops into bed at night. I told her that I can't stand being married to a lush, and I plan on leaving her. I've done everything in my power to get her to stop short of putting her in a cage, and I still can't get through to her. There is only one person who can help a hardcore alcoholic to become sober. They usually have to hit rock bottom to realize that they have a problem."

Sapphire's father didn't like hearing the truth about her, but he knew that every word that his son-in-law spoke was very true. After all, he had divorced Sapphire's mother because of her drinking problem. This severe alcoholism seemed to run in the family. She had an aunt who was also a lush. Rocky put up with a lot of crap in his life but was tired of tolerating life with an obsessive drunk.

A couple of times I remember being late when I had a secret meeting place set up to see Trudy. Once a customer of mine and his wife stopped by my house for a drink. I was late because they wanted to hang out, and I couldn't get them to leave, even though I was jittery and I looked at my watch every five minutes. Poor Trudy was alone at a restaurant for a long while without a car, not knowing if I was going to show or not. When I arrived, she told me that she was afraid that this relationship was not going to work out between us. She was tired of being the other woman. I couldn't blame her for having these feelings, but I felt this first love, high school kind of passion for her that I had never felt about any other woman. I couldn't stand the thought of losing her.

Then she hit me with a ton of bricks and said that she had an old boyfriend from Canada who was going to spend the weekend with her. Steve and Trudy were going to be together the entire time, enjoying each other's presence and mingling at the state fair. Of course, it scared me to death that there was a chance of losing her, so I demanded that he not come. Trudy got very upset and told me not to push her around and that she had to pursue her feelings toward Steve and see whether their relationship was really over or not. It was certainly unfair of me to expect Trudy to sit patiently and wait for me to decide when I was actually going to file for a divorce from Sapphire, but I've never liked losing to anyone or not getting my way, so this thing with Steve was hard for me to accept.

Practically from the minute that Steve stepped off his flight I remember her saying that this some-time-ago affair was probably going to come to a tragic halt—for Steve, anyway. You see, Trudy and I were able to see each other secretively that weekend without Steve having one clue to what was going on. She knew that she had allowed Steve to come that weekend more to get my dander up than to reevaluate her feelings about her old flame who was quickly becoming just a spark.

At first the hours spent with Steve away from me became torturous, the seconds ticking as slowly as if they were bogged down in heavy syrup. Trudy took advantage of any excuse that she could find to slip away from Steve to see me. I remember her roommate Linda having a dog that needed to be walked a lot—or at least she made it appear that way to Steve. In actuality, with every walk of that dog on the hour, she was really meeting up with me. I would be sitting on the curb a block down the street, waiting for her to fall into my arms and playing the tape of our favorite song, "Stuck on You" by Lionel Richie.

That weekend was simply going to be too long with Steve still in the picture, so I asked Trudy again to tell this guy to go back home. I remember her telling me that it wouldn't be right to say anything of that nature. He had spent a lot of cash on airfare and was expecting to go see the Alabama concert with her that night. I had to admit I loved her honesty, kindness, and sense of fairness. It was difficult to argue with Trudy because I knew she was right, so I told her to go to the concert with this jerk and then put an end to this old fling. I wanted him to be on a plane the next day and out of her life for good.

My teenage daughter Jennifer had been staying with Sapphire and me for the past year. Because she was very grown-up and wise for her age, I confided in her that I felt miserable knowing that Trudy was sharing her time with another man that weekend, even though I trusted her when she assured me that there was no further romantic interest in Steve. Jennifer told me that she had never seen me so obsessed with anything before, besides weightlifting, and she thought that I had lost my marbles. I remember her saying, "Dad, what's with you? You're acting nuts. I like Trudy, but come on. There are a lot of other women out there. Just forget about her. We'll go to the fair and have a great time, all right?" I wanted to take my daughter's advice and forget about Trudy for the moment, but I could not shake the thoughts of her in another man's arms.

Jennifer, a girlfriend of hers, and I all finally decided to head over to the fairgrounds. The three of us walked around for just a short while when I told the girls to go on ahead of me. Jennifer thought that I was getting a little stir crazy when I told her that I wanted to go look for my sweetheart. I didn't want to hold any of my feelings back any longer; I had to find her. My daughter said that I would never find her in that massive crowd, not knowing which one of the eight gates she would come out of. Jennifer was right: the odds of spotting Trudy would be about the same as seeing Jade, Ruby, and Sapphire all flocking out of the same exit together to greet me for coffee.

It could never happen, could it? I could never spot Trudy. Yet this driving force ran over every inch of logic as I told the girls that I would meet them back at the car at the stroke of midnight. I remember Jennifer rolling her eyes in a skyward direction and making it clear to me that she disapproved of my irrational behavior. She told me sarcastically to have fun sitting on a cold slab of concrete for the rest of the night.

I walked in a hurried fashion over to the pavilion, with the sound of Alabama's music getting louder with every step that I took. Once I arrived, I picked the first exit I saw, planted my rear end against a pillar, and waited. My eyes were frantically searching the entrance, praying that my true love would magically appear out of the pitch darkness.

Amazingly, within minutes my prayers had been answered because there she was, walking out of the auditorium alone. I rushed over to her and gave her the biggest bear hug imaginable. Then I looked at my sweet flower and said that I couldn't believe that I had found her so fast. My next instinct was to ask her what had happened. Trudy allowed her body the comfort and warmth of my embrace, hugging me tightly. She replied that she couldn't stand to be with Steve for one more second. He kept leaping all over her and wanted to hold hands like they were lovers. She finally couldn't take any more of it. At that very minute she shouted that she wanted to be with me, and I held her hand and said, "I will never let you go."

Fate certainly seemed to indicate that Rocky and Trudy were going to be companions for eternity. They were both still amazed that out of all the exits at the state fair pavilion, he had chosen the correct door. Trudy always felt bad about abandoning Steve like she had, despite his physical persistence. In fact, she called Steve in Canada, hoping to offer him a further apology, weeks after the state fair weekend. Trudy was never able to tell her former lover how sorry she was for the big misunderstanding. Steve pounded the receiver phone against its base, making her ears ring. So much for Trudy's apology.

Rocky had cheated on all three of his wives and really didn't care if he got caught. Trudy was not the reason he was going through another divorce; that had already been established because of Sapphire's drinking problem. At this point, Rocky could not even afford to hire an attorney because Sapphire had control of the family's money. He couldn't get his hands on their savings account because everything was in her name. Rocky had everything that all kids dream about: good looks, bulging muscles, over 150 trophies for his accomplishments, and an inspiring girlfriend…but no money! So Trudy loaned him $500 to put an end to his third marriage. Sapphire counter-served divorce papers and told her husband that he would be in the poorhouse once this was all over.

One day Rocky, his daughter Jennifer, Trudy, and her daughter decided to break into Rocky's own house. He wanted his prized possessions: his water bed (from a promotional deal), his toolbox, and of course his brass trophies. Jennifer broke through a side window to get in and unlock the front door. The first thing Trudy went for was his master bedroom closet. Trudy shouted, "Look what's in here, you guys! I just counted twenty-eight suit blazers and one silver fox coat probably worth over a grand." Then she gave Rocky the once over and said, "We're going shopping, my brave man. I can't believe a good-looking man like you lets your wife dress you in polyester suits with pointed collars. I don't want to have to call you Mr. Spock." She wanted to burn all his old clothes after she and Rocky picked out new ones, but he thought that they should at least go to the secondhand thrift store to get some cash for all his stuff.

"This stuff is junk," whispered the cashier to Trudy. "My boss won't let me even give you peanuts for this outdated clothing."

Trudy was very happy with her new muscleman's accomplishments and wanted him to look debonair and well-groomed. The fashionable couple rode down to New Orleans for the 1984 regular Mr. America Contest on an Amtrak with suitcases packed with fine threads but probably had four sawbucks and three fins between them, hidden deep in Trudy's purse. All of Rocky's paychecks went for Sapphire's $800 house payments and a nice place for the new couple to sleep when they were in town. At first they were as happy as two larks, singing and fellowshipping with strangers of different cultures from other parts of the country.

CHAPTER 9
MANAGING A RELATIONSHIP AND A BUSINESS COULD LEAD TO THE BOARDROOM

Sightseeing on the Amtrak was a great experience for the two lovebirds, something that neither would ever forget. There was also a third party involved on this trip down to New Orleans: Jennifer was invited to be a companion and to try to keep her dad out of mischief. As Rocky was looking out the window at the different terrains they were crossing over, he pondered the huge contest coming up. He knew that he would be competing against much younger and stronger body builders for the Mr. America pageant. Rocky knew that he was not in the best shape of his life like the previous year, but he still thought he had a chance at the title. At least this time the big man had two women at his side to help support him until the grand finale was over.

But then something came over Rocky all of a sudden. A young boy was running up and down the train aisle, being quite obnoxious. At that instant Rocky's mind snapped as he looked at Trudy and exploded, "I'd like to rip that kid's head off! Or maybe it should be the parent I should—"

Trudy interrupted by shouting back, "Your attitude is starting to suck, and if you don't straighten up, I'm going back home on another train. Come on, Jennifer. Let's go down to the dining car and have a drink." That was the sound of the raging steroids once again talking from the muscular man's framework.

At forty-two years of age in 1984, Rocky gave it his best shot but was not able to make it into the top fifteen contestants. He had numerous emotional setbacks gathering in his head afterward, but the one that stuck out the most in his mind was slightly overwhelming. After walking off the stage, Rocky thought, "What the hell am I doing to myself? I must be choking inside!" He assured Trudy and his daughter that he was not going to compete anymore and that he'd get off the sauce for good on the train ride home.

The next year, Rocky and Trudy decided to open their own weight training gym in Lake Geneva. She had always wanted her own business to manage, and he had the chance of a lifetime to get his workout sessions in and still make money. Rocky was able to get a $5,000 loan against his hog because that was the only thing that he owned of any significant value. Trudy also agreed to sink her life savings into the business, which the couple called the Weight Station. It was a very modern-looking gym with top-notch equipment. They eventually established a clientele of over 200 members. The business ran smoothly until the two-story building they were renting went up for sale. The business couple tried to buy the entire building so that they could live upstairs and not have to make payments on a house, but the building was finally sold to a dry-cleaning company, and Rocky and Trudy were given a sixty-day notice to pack their equipment and get out.

It didn't take them too long to find another building to rent on Highway H just south of Lake Geneva. The rent payments were three times more than they were in town. They eventually opened up a weight room and a juice bar in one of the large cubicles of this mini-mall location. Then they started aerobic classes in the adjoining cubicle to add some fun to their tedious workout schedule. About a month after the business started to take off, the city ripped up the highway, which seemed like indefinite construction.

The couple lost many of their customers because it was such a pain in the ass to get there and find parking. Trudy called Rocky into her office one day and said, "We need to go over our financial matters right now. We might have to file bankruptcy because we aren't making ends meet."

Rocky became aware of their financial status and said, "We're closing the gym." He knew quite a few gym owners and was able to sell their high-tech equipment for a good price. They actually made enough money from the sales to become debt-free. In the paperwork shuffle, Trudy and Rocky had never actually signed their lease for the building. The owner thought that he was out of luck until the couple personally presented the man with a check for over $2,000. He was simply amazed and confused at how anybody could be so honest. Rocky then moved all of the excess equipment into his basement for his own personal workout sessions. They closed that gym on December 31, 1985.

On a Sunday, January 5, 1986, Rocky and Trudy were at each other's throats while cleaning out their old gym office. They got into a huge verbal disagreement. "I used to work at this business from six o'clock in the morning until ten at night, pretty much taking care of the entire show. Then you would strut in after work, change into your gym attire, and be a prima donna."

"Well, I was in charge of getting some of our special programs together," answered Rocky.

"Yeah, you were in charge of showing off in front of all the cute babes that you brought in," replied Trudy. "I would get so pissed off while slaving behind my desk and watching you prance around half-naked, not showing one ounce of guilt!"

"You could have at least explained your feelings to me instead of walking out on me and the business that night," explained Rocky.

One night after work Rocky had seen a man behind the counter at the gym instead of Trudy. When he'd asked where Trudy was, the gentleman standing there had replied, "You don't want to know." He'd handed Rocky the notice that was on the door when he walked in that read: THIS BUSINESS IS CLOSED DUE TO LACK OF INTEREST, YOU CAN FIND ME AT THE BOARD-ROOM.

Mr. Adams had gone to get the key to let in Rocky's customers so they wouldn't miss out on any of their workouts. Rocky had been left in charge of his own gym and couldn't go out and look for Trudy until he was able to close up the business at 10:00 p.m. When he had finally gotten away, Rocky had advanced to the boardroom and found his girlfriend still there, a bit snookered up. When he'd spotted her, the big man had stopped dead in his tracks because he could almost see pitchforks in her eyes with smoke coming out of her ears. Rocky had said to himself, "Boy am I ever in trouble now!"

That night Rocky threw another one of his 'roid tantrums and brought the heel of his hand down on his Plymouth, which caved in the body corner where the windshield meets the roof about three-quarters of an inch. The body shop man said that was impossible to do because there was a steel bar underneath that corner for support. Wanting to prove to the guy that he had actually done it, Rocky tried to do the same thing on the opposite side and almost broke his hand. When you go into a steroid rage, you really never know the power of your own strength. Only the guy standing next to you does.

While still continuing to argue and bicker another evening, Trudy abruptly interrupted by asking Rocky a question that took him by surprise, "Will you go to church with me tonight?"

Rocky just hesitated and then laughed. He was speechless for the first time in years. Then he replied, "You've got to be out of your gourd. What do I want to go to church for? I haven't been to church in…I don't actually know how long it's been."

"Well, nothing seems to be going right between us, so maybe we should bring God into our relationship," answered Trudy.

"Where would you go to church at quarter to seven on a Sunday night?" asked Rocky.

"There's a Bible Church in Lake Geneva that I used to attend," answered Trudy. "It starts at 7:00 p.m."

"Just like a woman," Rocky mumbled. "But I'm in my sweat clothes. I need some time to—"

Trudy interrupted, "They don't care what you look like or how you dress."

The two of them hopped into their vehicle and drove down to the local church establishment for a different kind of spice in their lives. Having the huge ego that he did, Rocky sat in the front row pew by the center aisle. On top of that, he took off his sweatshirt with just a tank top underneath to show off his shoulder muscles. Rocky looked over at Trudy and spoke, "Don't expect me to listen to any sermons or take part in anything. I only came along because you asked me to."

The pastor spoke about people having problems and how they should accept Jesus Christ in their lives. He also mentioned "closet Christians" and how some people talk about doing one thing but actually do another, leading a hypocritical life. Rocky couldn't help but pay attention to this sermon, feeling as if this presentation were directed straight at him. The big man in sweats was so uplifted by the sermon that he turned to Trudy and asked, "Would you make a commitment with me? I would like for us to go to church together every Sunday this year." Trudy was definitely stunned by that response, but she agreed to acknowledge Rocky's request. "I believe that we do need a change in our lives. There aren't too many things going right for me: the eternal string of divorces, losing the business…this is all taking a heavy toll."

"Keep your voice down to a low roar," interrupted Trudy. "Stop talking and listen to what the pastor is saying."

Another fifteen minutes of the sermon went by and Rocky inched closer to his girlfriend and whispered, "I want you to do me a favor. Let's think about dedicating our lives to Christ. Perhaps that'll change my life around."

The couple went to church the following Sunday and were greeted at the front door. "How are you doing on this fine Sunday morning?"

Rocky answered, "It's funny you asked that because I have a knack for breaking records."

The greeter asked, "And how's that?" thinking that this huge man might be off his rocker or something.

Rocky snickered and said, "Well, this is our second Sunday of this new year already to attend church. You see, I only went once last year."

Eleven days after the couple appeared in the front pew that Sunday night, Rocky was being prepped for surgery. A golf ball-sized lump had appeared out of nowhere when he was shaving off his beard about a week before. Trudy had him call their doctor at the Burlington Clinic to be checked out. The doctor explained that it was a thyroidal cyst that needed to come out. It was near the lymph node area, and it could give him a problem or cause an infection.

Rocky had a one-day surgery scheduled for January 16. After lunch that day, Trudy and her girlfriend Linda were coming back from lunch and thought Rocky would be back in his recovery room by then. He was in his designated room all right, but to stay for a while longer.

"The tests came back from pathology, and I'm afraid you have a malignant lymph node," stated Rocky's doctor.

Rocky asked, "What does that mean?"

The surgeon answered, "Rocky, I have some bad news to tell. You have cancer."

Rocky looked up toward the ceiling and thought, "Is this problem from my steroid usage, Lord?"

A suspicious-looking character wearing a trench coat entered the main doorway to Trudy and Rocky's Weight Station gym, carrying a leather bag in his hand. Trudy caught on to this guy right away and knew what was going on. Rocky had sworn to her that he was not going to indulge in the steroid habit anymore after the 1984 Mr. America contest. Trudy walked up to this character and screamed in his ear, "The substance you have in that duffle bag, my friend, we don't even have in our vocabulary in this establishment. You need to take your swinging drugstore as far away from here as you can get, or I'll have the cops on your ass before you can say, 'Please, Sheriff Taylor, tell that deputy of yours not to feed the jail cell key to his pet goat.'"

"I'm leaving, lady. Don't call anybody, please," answered the stranger.

Meanwhile, Rocky pulled up into the parking lot of the gym after work. Trudy happened to look out the window to see this character making physical contact with her man. She heard them talking as Rocky forked over some American cash for German Dianabol steroids that the guy had in his bag. Trudy decided that she would play along with this little charade.

A few days later, Trudy was coming home from running errands and headed straight for the bathroom. Much to her surprise, she was not alone. Instead, she witnessed an experience that she would never forget. She caught Rocky in the act, with his pants down, staring at a syringe sticking out of his right buttock. He was giving himself an injection.

She spoke out with flaming features, "This relationship is over. This is final. I'm out of here!" Trudy went over to her girlfriend's house to spend the night.

An hour or so later, Rocky called to tell Trudy that he had flushed all the steroids down the toilet and didn't even finish the one she saw in his ass. She did not believe him for one instant. Trudy let her disgraced man sleep on this situation but went back over in the morning to pay him a visit.

"I can't take this anymore. I really can't, Rocky," expressed Trudy. "I will not spend the rest of my life with someone who I might have to take care of for the rest of his." The surge of power that Rocky would get after shooting up would not be tolerated by the woman who still loved him deeply. She wanted him to have that feeling about their lives together without the use of drugs. In her eyes, her man was digging himself a six-foot-deep hole. Trudy decided to give Rocky one more chance to cooperate with her perspective of how life should be, otherwise she would be gone forever.

The couple confided in Bob Goldwin, who did all the steroid testing for the Olympics. Bob quoted from experience, "If you lower your immune system by the use of steroids the possibility of triggering dormant cancer cells increases at an incredible rate." The last injection that Rocky actually did finish sped up his metabolism, which created his golf ball-sized lump.

Trudy suggested that they get a second opinion. They went to the Cancer Research Department at the University of Wisconsin Hospital in Madison. The physician in charge presented Rocky and Trudy with the true medical facts. "Your other doctor was right on the money. Without treatment, you have less than ninety days to live. So I suggest we take one step at a time. Let's try to cure this unfortunate situation, which is in stage IV."

"What does this mean?" asked Rocky.

"Well, you do have a chance of beating this, if you start treatment right away," explained the doctor.

Rocky's brother Charlie and his wife were also at his bedside trying to figure out this horrible situation. "Is this hereditary, doctor?" asked Charlie.

Trudy could not even believe that question was asked. Her sweetheart Norman was just given a diagnosis with possibly only a short time to live. All Charlie was worried about was himself.

The physician in charge spoke, "Yes, cancer is hereditary. But Rocky, you can count your blessings that you did that last steroid shot. We feel that you've had cancer for about six months now, but without detecting that lump, you probably would not have come in for a checkup. This type of cancer could have spread to all of your major organs within a short period of time."

Trudy answered, "Well, I guess we can thank the good Lord and Rocky's way of thinking for that."

The doctor went on to say, "We have an experimental program that is just starting. This might be a good chance for you. The physicians involved are going to start treating 200 people with this new type of medicine that has been approved. Would you like for me to see if there are any more openings?"

Trudy asked, "Doctor, in this same situation with your family, would you be able to make a decision like this?"

The doctor answered, "Yes, I would. These new drugs have been tested, and it is my opinion that they're going to be rated highly. I have a lot of confidence in this."

It turned out that there was exactly one opening left. Without hesitation, Rocky said, "I'll take it."

The first large dose of this toxic medication took about an hour or so for the nurse to administer. Rocky could feel the warmth in his veins, which left a terrible taste in his mouth, after the poison was injected. Since the side effects could be quite drastic, the physician wanted Rocky's condition to be monitored throughout the night. Trudy spent the night there on a cot near her man's side. Rocky stayed awake practically all night, just watching the time gradually tick away.

The next morning his doctor briefly checked in on him with all of his interns following closely behind. "How do you feel this morning, Mr. Rauch?"

Rocky answered, "I feel great. Can somebody around here get me some breakfast?"

The doctor replied, "You're hungry? I'll have someone get on that request immediately." Two hospital trays with double helpings of food were brought in, and every last crumb was devoured. The doctors were very surprised that Rocky had not felt sick at all during the night.

The divorce proceedings between Rocky and Sapphire were coming closer to a halt. He was able to keep the insurance from her job for eighteen months by law. When the insurance was no longer available, Rocky would have to transfer over to the VA hospital wing to continue his treatment. It was actually an adjoining building where he could continue treatment with the same physician and staff.

Through this program it was mandatory for Rocky to receive chemotherapy every twenty-eight days. He would still work at his job except for the day of his treatment and the day after. Some days Trudy would drive him around to deal with customers so he could rest in between stops.

During treatment Rocky didn't know how much more of this life on earth he could take. People would even look at him strangely because of his hair loss. A profit of $28,000 was earned on the house that he and Sapphire owned together. She received $14,000, and the remaining $14,000 also was awarded to her because of his pension plan debt to her. Rocky did not think that was fair, but at least he didn't owe any money to anybody.

In total, Rocky had lost his gym business, his three gems, and his wavy locks, and he didn't know if he would live or die. But Rocky kept his faith, and with Trudy always by his side, he somehow got by. Sapphire never called once to see how Rocky was doing with his treatments.

Finally all those memories were put to rest. Rocky was still hanging on by a thread, which in time turned into a thick braided rope. He was tugging away as hard as possible to win his battle against cancer. Rocky went through many months of chemotherapy, and just when he felt that he was getting stronger, he heard that his boss had the opportunity to sell the business. Rocky was eventually notified that his company was being sold. His boss called to apologize and to tell him that the new ownership probably wouldn't keep him.

The pastor of their church was invited over for lunch one day before the divorce was finalized with Sapphire. "How long have you been married?" asked the pastor.

Rocky hesitated and looked over at Trudy. "Oh, we aren't married. We're just living together."

"Well, I can tell you this much," explained the pastor. "'Living together' is not tolerated in our church. You are living in sin, and you must join hands in matrimony in order to become full-fledged members of our congregation."

"But we can't get married," replied Rocky. "I'm still going through a divorce with my third wife."

That statement threw the pastor for a loop. He then hesitated, and replied, "I'll check with the members of the council and try to get funding for Trudy to live elsewhere."

Rocky and Trudy decided to live separately because it was the right thing to do. It was the Lord's way. Rocky felt as if he really needed Christ in his life, especially now. Trudy looked for a roommate to share expenses and help with the rent, and eventually she met a girl who basically had the same intentions. Laurie and Trudy became best of friends, and Laurie gave her life to Christ also.

Instead of depression, Rocky built his confidence and self-esteem back up and proposed marriage to Trudy. She hesitated and told Rocky that she didn't want to answer that question with a positive answer until he was feeling much better and all of his treatments and therapy were over. Trudy wanted to marry Rocky for love and an everlasting relationship and not for sympathy. She also mentioned that if he ever gave her another proposal, it most certainly had to be at a special place—not McDonald's or Burger King, and not in the car.

Rocky took on another job with a swimming pool company out of Chicago as a sales representative. They knew that he was still going through therapy but still wanted to hire him because of his reputation with the last company he worked for. One night at the Arlington Heights Hilton Hotel, a gathering of important people from the company showed up for a meeting and show and to dine in the evening. The dining hall was elegant, with violin players and chandeliers. Rocky said to himself, "This certainly isn't McDonalds. Maybe I should ask Trudy that important question for the second time." The big man lowered himself to the red carpet on one knee exactly when the string quartet ended their piece. "Will you marry me, Trudy?" You could have heard a pin drop at that moment.

Trudy started to shed some tears but did not react with an answer to her man's question immediately. The well-dressed associates at the table started to make comments, "Come on. Rocky's waiting desperately for an answer. If his leg falls asleep, he'll never get up."

The surrounding fan club started to chant, "We want an answer! We demand an answer right now!"

The waitresses standing behind the couple commented, "This has never happened before."

Trudy wiped away her tears and smiled. "Yes, I will marry you." At that moment, the entire place went into an uproar.

Champagne, compliments of the house, was brought to their table, and one of the executives stood up and shouted, "I will pay for a honeymoon suite for this happy couple to spend the night. You two are not driving all the way back to Lake Geneva."

The next morning, the owner of Rocky's new place of employment spotted the engaged couple walking down a flight of stairs. "I thought that you went home last night," he said. "I guess that I might have missed something?"

Grinning from ear to ear, Rocky replied, "I proposed to Trudy last night at our table. We will announce our wedding date very soon."

The owner asked, "Does this mean that you are...?"

"Yes, sir, I am in remission now, which means that I completely licked my cancer," interrupted Rocky. His head boss was elated to hear the fantastic news.

Rocky and Trudy were pronounced husband and wife on June 27, 1987. The pastor who presented the sermon that first Sunday night when the couple sat in the front pew married them. The splendid wedding and reception were held in the high school gymnasium. The couple was escorted there in a burgundy Xcaliber sports car that matched Rocky's tuxedo. Rocky's brother stood up for him, and Trudy's daughter was the maid of honor. The attending friends and relatives, especially the ones who knew of Rocky and Trudy's background, expected to have a grand time at the wedding. It turned out to be an unannounced dry wedding, with no booze allowed on the premises.

The couple spent their honeymoon together at the Wisconsin Dells, where they started their brand new Christian life together as a married, jubilant couple.

Rocky continued to work for the Mallhawk Pool Corporation and reached $1 million in sales in the first year. He was promised 5% sales commission if he supplied his own transportation and paid most of the expenses. The only competition was his former company, which basically had sales routes in the same general locations. Rocky never said anything bad about his old company for letting him go. If the customers would ask, he would just tell them that it was time to make a change in his life when his former pump and spa company changed ownership. Instead of making $50,000 his first year, the leading salesman made about half that. Their concept was that if you sold everything at catalog price, then you would get the 5% commission. A legal binding contract was never signed by either party.

It worked out that Rocky basically received 2.5% sales commission while supplying his own transportation and paying expenses. He felt cheated, and he put feelers out to look for another job. A lady by the name of Pearl gave Rocky a buzz on the telephone one day and asked about his health and his job. He explained that he was in remission and felt fine, but his job wasn't going toward his liking. Rocky used to sell this lady's line of bath tubs when he was with the old pump company. Pearl told Rocky that she would personally call him back if there were any openings in her company. Months went by, but he didn't hear a thing from her.

Eventually Pearl contacted Rocky again and said that she wanted a sales representative for the state of Wisconsin. So Trudy and her husband drove up to Minneapolis so he could be interviewed by Pearl's son John. The interviewer was impressed with Rocky's background, and Pearl was fascinated by Trudy's personality. The executives from that division met that week, and Rocky was offered a job with a base salary plus commission. The two parties negotiated, and Rocky, being the salesman that he was, squeezed a little more out of them to satisfy his wallet.

Rocky was hired to go to work for Pearl and her bath and spa company on April 1 of the year after their marriage. On that same date, which was Good Friday, Rocky waited around for hours to receive his last commission check from Mallhawk. After receiving his check, he handed in his resignation papers and said that he officially started with another company that day.

"This must be an April Fool's joke," stated one of the executives.

"No joke," explained Rocky. "This is everything I've been dreaming about. I'm going to be a regional manager in the state of Wisconsin. It will be another stepping stone to move forward on in my life."

Rocky had an illustrious career with Pearl's company for seven years.

A loud doorbell ring was heard from Rocky's front porch one day when he was home still going through chemotherapy. A young teenager was standing near the threshold. As the door swung open, the kid spoke in a determined manner, "Can you tell me where Rocky's Gym is at?"

Rocky hesitated and replied, "We don't have a gym anymore, son. At one time we owned the Weight Station here in town, but that's been closed for some time now."

The high school kid introduced himself and also said, "I work out at the YMCA in town, but I'm getting frustrated. Nobody there really wants to help me. I just heard that you're really good at weight training and might be able to give me some pointers."

Rocky answered, "I'm sorry, kid, but I have some problems of my own right now. I really can't help you."

The boy gleamed into the big man's eyes and said, "I really want to work out."

Rocky thought for a moment and then invited the kid inside, "Why don't you come with me." The young boy followed him down a flight of stairs into a section of his own personal basement gym. The equipment left over from the Weight Station, plus Rocky's collection of older weights from when he started, were all set up.

"This is really neat," the kid blurted out.

The downstairs gym actually had a ground level door with a lock and a bathroom with a shower. Showing the kid around, started the wheels turning in Rocky's mind. "How would you like to work out here, kid?" asked Norman.

The kid spoke up instantly, "That would be fantastic!"

For $10 a month, this eager high school teenager had acquired his own personal key and a weight program to follow, made up by the one and only 1983 Mr. America champion. What more could a kid ask for?

This was the beginning of Rocky's private Key Club Gym, open to all honest kids and pastors. By word of mouth, this growing little business became Rocky's second family that helped to support him through his time of need.

CHAPTER 10
DOWN ON HIS LUCK AGAIN

Things seemed to be going a little smoother for Rocky and his wife Trudy, with their second family of kids stopping by to visit the basement Key Club Gym. This was one of Rocky's desires: to help teach the younger generation a few tricks of the trade. Since he wasn't in the limelight much anymore, Rocky wanted to see the youth of the future progress and make something out of themselves. Trudy would converse with the boys about girlfriend problems or whatever they might want to talk about on their breaks. She would also have good protein snacks for them. It was 1988, with snow on its way soon and people getting into the holiday spirit. The couple had a trip to Florida all planned out after Rocky's next cancer checkup.

Dr. Stone at the Burlington Hospital went through the normal procedure to do the follow-up. After examining the lymph nodes in his neck and armpits, the physician could tell that there was something wrong. "I hate to be the one to tell you this, Rocky," explained Dr. Stone, "but your cancer is back. I'm not sure how bad it is at this time. We'll have to do some testing in the near future, with your permission, of course, but I want you to do one thing for me before we start your series of tests."

"What's that, doc?" asked Rocky.

"I want you and your wife Trudy to take that vacation that you have been talking about," replied the doctor.

The couple did what the doctor ordered and went to Florida to visit Trudy's parents. They also wanted serenity to be alone and share their love. The perfect couple tried not to think about the inevitable future. What was in store for the man who had thought he was starting to get his life back on track? Would he live or would he die? The two-week stay in Florida was very difficult for both Rocky and Trudy.

Dr. Stone arranged for Rocky to go through the cancer testing once again when he arrived back home. A bone marrow biopsy was performed, and the doctor explained that the cancer had not spread as far as it had the first time. An oral pill was out on the market that would make his chemotherapy much easier to take. The side effects were not nearly as bad compared to what the injections were like for most people. So Rocky was given the instructions to do the chemo for three weeks on and then one week off. This took place over a six-month period.

On one of his road trips, Rocky stopped off at a small hometown diner for lunch. He removed his cap, which exposed his bald head, and put it on the seat next to him. A young high school waitress asked him what he would like to order and then walked back to talk with her peers. He noticed the girls staring and giggling in the background. Sometimes he felt self-conscious of his baldness, mainly because he did not want people to feel sympathetic toward his condition.

The young waitress hurried back over to her table and asked a favor, "Can I get your autograph, sir?"

Rocky immediately started to snicker and answered, "Why would you want my autograph?"

"Well, I see you on professional wrestling every Saturday morning," the waitress replied.

Rocky let out a loud laugh, but he could understand why he was mistaken for a huge muscular wrestler. He weighed approximately 240 pounds with a bald head, and he had that ringmaster type of look. Still smiling at the waitress, Rocky humbly spoke out, "I lost my hair because I'm going through chemotherapy for the second time. I was on steroids for many years to enhance my body-building career, which I am not proud of. But I am proud of winning the Mr. America title back in 1983. Now if you still want my autograph, I would be honored to give it to you."

The young girl smiled back and said, "That would totally make my day. I have a boyfriend who likes to work out a lot. Sometimes I think that he loves that more than he loves me."

"I totally can understand that. Believe me," Rocky answered.

"My boyfriend will be happy to know that I had the opportunity to meet you, sir," replied the waitress.

"Just call me Rocky, young lady," stated Rocky.

"I just hope that my boyfriend isn't thinking about using steroids, Rocky," said the girl. The word spread within a few minutes that they had a celebrity in the house, and he ended up signing napkins, pant legs, a guy's bald head...whatever the workers and customers in the café wanted.

After that scene, Rocky put his cap away for good and never wore one again while going through his chemo. If he looked like a professional wrestler to some people, then that was cool enough for him. The muscular man still had an incentive to work out in his own basement gym. He could still bench press 350 pounds of massive iron weights. The doctors said that he could lift weights to keep in shape as long as he took it easy. Rocky didn't know the meaning of the words TAKE IT EASY. If there was no pain, then there would be no gain.

When Rocky's kids saw him going through chemo and still bench pressing a ton of weight, that inspired them to work all that much harder. And watching the boys give every ounce of strength in striving to be the best was a huge uplift and encouragement for Rocky. A little flavor was added to the work-out sessions when Rocky would say such things like, "Watch this, guys. When I move my head from side to side, I look like the roll-on deodorant with eyes from that cartoon commercial."

After his six months of chemo, Rocky's cancer was eliminated, and he went back into remission. Dr. Stone said that he would be a good candidate for a bone marrow transplant. He also explained to Rocky that since his cancer had come back again within a five-year period, the chances of it happening a third time were high.

In the meantime, Rocky was asked to be a speaking candidate for a women's fashion show. It was a ladies' luncheon with over 800 women present. Top athletes and their wives from the Green Bay Packers, Milwaukee Brewers, and Milwaukee Bucks were there to model clothes for this gigantic fundraiser. The theme for the children's cancer research project was "Run the Race to Win." All the television station cameras were focused on Rocky as he was speaking from his heart, "You know, when you see all these young kids in the hospital, some bald from chemo at the early age of three or four, you just can't help but get a little bit emotional. It's like the message in that TV commercial: everyone just needs to reach out and touch someone."

After Rocky's speech, all 800 women were in tears, and they stood up and gave him a standing ovation. He never claimed to be an orthodox speaker who always used the correct pronouns and adjectives in his sentences, but he got the message across and received many compliments from all of the news commentators there.

A short time later Rocky read in the USA TODAY newspaper about how they were announcing an 800-number to call and talk to highly-rated physicians on steroid abuse for the next three days. This was fantastic news to the man who knew more about steroids affecting people's lives than anybody. He dialed that telephone number and got a hold of a woman who he thought was just a customer service person. "Hello. My name is Norman Rauch, and I just wanted to commend you on that well-written article and how you are allowing people like me to give our views on steroid abuse," explained Rocky.

"Why are you so interested, Mr. Rauch?" asked the head sports editor.

"Well, I'm a former steroid abuser," informed Rocky. "They almost took my life. I almost died from cancer."

"Why did you take the steroids?" asked the sports editor.

"You see, I'm a former Mr. America—"

"What?" interrupted the lady. "You are a former Mr. America who was abusing steroids and you are calling in regards to our article? Where are you?"

"I'm in Philadelphia for one more day," answered Rocky. "But tomorrow I'm leaving for Allentown to visit my mother. I have a speaking engagement there at my old high school. An old workout buddy of mine is a teacher there and wants me to speak on steroid abuse because he suspects it's going on with athletes at the high school."

"We need to set up a time to interview you and get a full story," replied the sports editor. "It's unbelievable that you are calling us."

"Well, I'm not doing this for a story about myself," said Rocky. "I'm just calling to say that this is a great thing that you're doing, getting this topic out of the closet."

The editor would not take no for an answer. She spoke in a forceful manner, "Could you please give me a phone number for where you can be reached? Also, is there a gym near your mom's home?"

"Yeah, I have a friend who owns a gym there," explained Rocky. "That's where I'll be working out during my stay in Allentown. Why?"

"I'd like to send some professional photographers there," replied the sports editor, "and do a photo shoot of you working out."

Rocky decided to let *USA Today* do their photo session and newspaper article just for one main reason: to speak out to all young athletes throughout the world on how harmful steroids can be to the human body. The sports writer who interviewed Rocky for the story said that the article would appear on the front page on October 28, 1988, the day he was scheduled to speak at his old high school. The MORNING CALL hometown newspaper that Norman was a carrier for in his childhood days, also wanted to put out a story.

A couple of days before Rocky's speaking engagement, the school principal called to say that he wanted to cancel the event.

Only fifteen kids had signed up to be there. Rocky was bound and determined to reach out to any young athlete he could possibly get through to. He told the principal that he still wanted to give the presentation even if only two kids showed up.

On the morning of the 28th, both newspapers kept their promises and featured Rocky with his story and photo on the front page. Over 300 kids showed up for his high school presentation. This was the first time that Rocky had ever given a speech at a local high school, and he gave one of the best performances of his life. He thought that if he was able to get through to one kid, it would have made his job worthwhile. As Rocky was getting ready to leave the auditorium, a young teenage boy approached him and thanked him for giving that great talk on steroid abuse.

The kid started to explain, "Mr. Rauch, I learned a whole lot today from you. My buddies are doing the drugs and are trying to talk me into doing them also. After I heard what you are going through, I don't want any part of this steroid scene. If I'm going to make it in this sports business, I'm going to do it without 'a little help from my friends.'" Rocky reached over and gave the kid the biggest bear hug imaginable.

A few days after Rocky arrived back home in Wisconsin, the ESPN sports station did a phone interview and a photo session with him that was going to air the following Saturday. He was starting to get nationwide attention after the front page article came out in *USA Today*. Rocky also received a call to do "The Today Show" out in Seattle, Washington, with the mother of a boy named Michael Keys.

For Michael, it had started at the age of 15. He worked out in his basement while depending on oral steroids. His goal was to become big and strong, not really to compete in physical contact sports. The drug started to affect him in mysterious ways. One minute he could be in a serene mood, and the next he might be having a steroid rage. It was like Dr. Jekyll and Mr. Hyde. One morning Michael tried to open his car door, but the lock was frozen stuck from the cold climate. So he continued to try and rip the door apart with his own physical strength. Not succeeding at that,

Michael ran back into the house and trashed his bedroom from wall to wall. Then he went down into the basement, crawled into a sleeping bag, put a .22 rifle to his chin, and blew himself away. Michael had taken his own life at the young age of 17 because of the affects that steroids can have on your emotional state of mind.

After the excitement from the news and sports stations died down a bit, Rocky took some time off to be a bone marrow transplant candidate. A few months into the new year, he had to go through a strict series of extensive testing to make sure this procedure could be performed. The physicians thoroughly checked out every part of this man's physical anatomy. The testing procedures lasted for two days. Some things were borderline, but Rocky's physician in charge announced, "Your bone marrow is cancer-free at this time. This is what I'd like to suggest. We think that this would be the perfect time to harvest it."

"Please explain why you would want to do that," stated Rocky.

"Since your bone marrow is free from cancer," replied the physician, "we can eject it from your body and freeze it with liquid nitrogen. You would become your own donor. It would have a ten-year shelf life, and we can always inject it back into your system if your cancer comes back." The doctor went on to explain to Trudy, "This would be the best scenario because Rocky's physiological system would theoretically never reject his own donation, whereas if he depended upon a brother or a daughter, for instance, there could be complications down this rocky road. That should never be ruled out."

Rocky and Trudy decided, with the expert advice of the specialists, to go through with this operation. Rocky would have to give up three pints of blood over a three-week period at the Milwaukee Blood Center (where Sapphire still worked), for his harvest. He would be set up to be his own donor.

Then came the rough part of the bone marrow procedure. The experts would extract three liters of bone marrow out of Rocky's hip bone with a giant syringe. They would make a one-inch incision in the bone and do approximately 200 aspirations. The tissue around the bone could be frozen, but the surgeons couldn't actually numb the bone marrow itself because it is a liquid. It turned out to be a very painful and costly operation.

In December of 1989, Rocky was given the news that he did not want to hear. His third round of cancer cells had distinctively made another appearance.

Although Rocky had six speaking engagements at high schools coming up, the number-one specialist on his case wanted to do the bone marrow transplant as soon as possible. In order to keep the cancer from spreading any further, it was mandatory that they perform the transplant immediately. Rocky was given a 60 percent chance of possibly beating this dreadful enemy for the third time.

Rocky had one last opportunity to speak at the Hartford High School the day before his bone marrow transplant operation. The principal of the school was given the message that he was going to present himself in front of the students with a Mohawk. The authoritative figure begged Rocky not to make an appearance like that. He gave the big man an earful, "I know that my students are going to think that you are the coolest guy to ever hit their high school, but if you show up like that tomorrow, the next day all of my students will look like *The Last of the Mohicans!*"

Statistics showed that out of 20,000 people there would be one match for a bone marrow transplant. At the time, there were over 11,000 others waiting on that one perfect match. Rocky and Trudy both felt that the frozen bone marrow in the bank was more than a gift from heaven. It was a security blanket that would be a great blessing in saving the big man's life.

On January 29, 1990, Rocky checked into the Milwaukee County Medical Hospital for treatment. He had prepared himself for this transplant just as he would have for an ordinary weightlifting competition. His bodyweight had been beefed up to a healthy 250 pounds of solid muscle. He felt that the stronger he was, the better the chance of him staying in this world. But the truth was that he had no inclination of what was in store for him in the near future.

Since he hated hospital clothes, Rocky packed two suitcases full of psychedelic sweatshirts and pants. There was an assortment of crazy colors with handprints, zebra stripes, and leopard spots painted all over them. He wanted to brighten up his hospital floor by wearing his *Back to the Future* sunglasses and showing off his Mohawk haircut.

When Rocky arrived at the nurses' station dressed like a being from another planet, he pounded his fist down on the counter and asked, "Where's my room?"

All the nurses on duty stopped dead in their tracks. It was just like someone had pressed the pause button on the hospital's TV remote. The head nurse asked, "Who are you?"

"I am the Rock. I have arrived!" exclaimed Rocky, trying to put a little color back into this picture.

The nurses on the floor thought that this guy was completely out of his gourd. Rocky thought for a moment that they were all going to point to the sign hanging from the ceiling to direct him to the Psychiatric Ward. It turned out that most of the nurses were fighting and bickering amongst themselves to see who would be taking care of this unique man.

The room that Rocky was assigned to had an air-flow system that was germ-free. Every fifth day a plumber would come in to replace the shower heads because of germ contamination. Rocky had to be fitted with a special denture mold that was filled with a certain gel to keep the germs away. He also had to swallow a giant pill that would prevent any mouth sores from accumulating. Since his immune system was going to be lowered immensely, the hospital attendants had to use every precautionary method available to keep the room spotless and clear of any type of germs.

The following words from the heart explain what Rocky did not foresee coming into his life when he was training to become the strongest man alive. Who could know the facts about his three bouts with cancer and the inviting encounters with death more than his dependable and sacrificing wife Trudy? She was there for him, God bless her!

This is Trudy's story, told in her own words:

ROCKY'S ROAD

As I look back I wonder how I got through it all. Back in 1984 I met a man who was 6' 3" 230 pounds and all muscle. After all, he won Mr. America 1983 and he was in shape. Little did I know he would pay the price for all those muscles later. During our relationship I found out that he did anabolic steroids. Until he started doing steroids again in 1985 I knew nothing about them, but believe me I found out quite quick what they did to him...they made him very aggressive... he wasn't the Rocky I first met. It turned him into a jerk...a me, myself, and I; wearing muscle shirts and wanting everyone to notice him. Believe me they did. I at first thought it was cool to be with a guy so good looking and a body and brains to match. At 42 years old, he was very successful in the business world. What more could a woman want...little did I know that I would fall in love with him, and marry him. This is where true love comes, when your boyfriend is told (Jan. 1986) that he has non-Hodgkin Lymphoma and less than 90 days to live. Wow, am I hearing the doctor right? Cancer. It is only my love for the Lord and love for Rocky that kept me at his side. He was on extensive chemo for 10 months and never got sick. He did get very tired and did not have a lot of energy. So, I quit my job to drive him around. He is a salesman and on the road a lot. He only lost two days a month, the day of his treatment and the day after. The cancer went into remission after about 10 months for around 2 years. We were married on June 27, 1987.

Rocky felt that he had to get into the schools to tell them about steroids...but the schools said they didn't have a problem with that. Rocky had problems and had tests done earlier in his weightlifting career. He was seen by a doctor who told him that it was the steroids that were causing his problems. He had a breakout of boils all over his body. Rocky was told that if he wanted to live a fruitful life, he would have to quit the steroids before it killed him. The doctors won't say, "Yes, steroids caused his cancer", but they do say that the steroids caused an immune system breakdown that allowed the cancer to become more aggressive. Rocky describes it as playing Russian Roulette with your life. It couldn't happen to me, you might say. Well in Rocky's case it did, and if he could do it all over again knowing what he would have to go through, he would tell you it is not worth it. There is a price to pay for everything we do somewhere in our life. Well, since then Rocky has gotten the message out to schools, colleges, anyone who would listen.

In 1988 his cancer came back. He was treated for 24 weeks and it went back into remission. At that time our doctor suggested that we see if Rocky was eligible for a bone marrow transplant. They did a lot of tests including a double bone marrow biopsy, and found out that he was cancer free. Toward the end of the year, they put him in the hospital and did his harvest. The good Lord was looking over him to give him another chance for life. Getting a bone marrow transplant is like getting a new life, only Rocky gave himself his own new life. Most cancer patients don't have a chance to do that; there new life might come from a sibling, or otherwise they have only a 1 in a 20,000 chance for an outside match. There are over 11,000 people waiting for a match...or another chance for a new life. My prayer for those waiting for a match, is that someone like you might want to call the local blood center to find out how to give a new life to someone. Just think, it could be you or a family member, or a friend that is waiting. The more people that are typed, the better the chances of the people waiting will be. Well, Rocky now has his bone marrow frozen, but we hope and pray that he will never use it.

We were ready for a vacation to Florida once again. Rocky had an appointment with the doctor before we left. "I don't want to tell you this before you leave, but I need to, your cancer is back. You will be okay to take your trip...go and have a good time and forget everything until you come back. At that time we will discuss your transplant."

Well, we went on our trip teary eyed, but it was the best trip we ever had together. I guess it was the fear of not knowing if we would ever have the chance to have another trip together. Neither one of us talked about that, but as I look back, I am sure that it crossed both of our minds. We had a special time with our Lord and put our minds on top of things and away from any negative thoughts. We knew with the Lord's help, Rocky would win. He had himself so prepared for the transplant...even down to what he would wear when he was in the hospital. He said he was going to brighten the floor up when he got there...well he did with his wild and crazy colored clothing and hats.

Then came admission, with the first 3 days of tests, tests, and more tests. Day one was the start of chemo, three times a day for three days. This was not fun for Rocky...first you get sick and the side effects from the chemo are bad, then they give you more drugs to combat the side effects. By the fourth day that they say is your rest day, believe me, Rocky did anything but rest. They got him up three times a day to take a stroll in the hall...bone marrow patients call it the bone marrow shuffle...you have all you can do to put one foot in front of the other while you push your IV pole in front of you. We called the IV pole Rocky's Robot as it was stacked high with three pumps that gave him his meds. I can't say enough about all the care Rocky got from the doctors and nurses. As I watched other bone marrow transplant patients, I thought some had an easier time than others, but believe me, none of them really have it easy. As Rocky was getting the treatments, they would come in and tell me step by step what would happen. One thing they do is catheterize patients, because the chemo is so strong, that it could burn a hole in their bladder. They give them an IV flush. Rocky looked forward to the day of rest when they took the catheter out. Then the fifth day comes along and they tell you that for the next three days, they will be giving you total body radiation, three times a day for twenty minutes at a time. Now you can see the chemo going in, but there is something about not knowing what the radiation will do...and then they tell you about all the side effects that can happen. I mean to tell you that this is scary, and I had a hard time dealing with the unknown.

Back on test day I remember them making lead blocks in the shape of Rocky's major organs, that would protect him from the radiation. Well on day one they made him dress in a hat, gown, gloves, mask, and took him down to x-ray where they put him in a concrete room with two lead doors. He was propped up on a bicycle seat with a seat belt to help give him some support. There was this huge Plexiglas shield in front of him which they called a splash shield. At that time everyone had to leave the room. The lead doors closed and the radiation was administered while I watched Rocky on a TV monitor, crying my eyes out. I was able to talk to him over a sound system and all I could say was, "I love you." It tore my heart out. The feeling is unexplainable, unless you go through it all, you could never know. By the time you get to the last day, the last treatment, you can barely stand, or for that matter even want to. I think that at this point most patients don't care, don't remember. Rocky was ready to cash in. It was the only time I had ever known him to just want to quit, or just plain lie down and die. It's remarkable how the Lord's timing is perfect...just as Rocky said, "I just want to die," a nurse comes in wheeling a crib with a baby girl in it who had a Hickman catheter in place. She was an 18 month old girl with leukemia going in for radiation. Ya see, she didn't have a choice. Rocky saw her and with tears in his eyes said, "If she can do it so can I." I thank God for his timing. As I watched him go through his last radiation treatment I asked myself, "What is happening?" If this can kill cancer cells and damage your vital organs, what in the world is it doing to his brain? And will he be okay? When you're all stressed out, it is just amazing what our minds can think of. That's where my faith in the Lord kept me sane, and gave me just what I needed to get through this. Then comes the seventh day and you receive your new life. Some families celebrate a new life with a birthday party. And that is just what we did. I had some special people in Rocky's room to celebrate his new birthday.

Rocky was now going to use his own bone marrow that was frozen in liquid nitrogen. They would thaw out 2 syringes at a time and administer it into his Hickman which goes into the main artery of the heart. There were 8 syringes and it took about 4 hours to get it all in. As I watched and prayed, I asked God for the miracle of a new life. The people on the bone marrow floor have a special bond with each other. There are times when you support each other by praying and sometimes crying together. At the time of the bone marrow transplant, Rocky's white count was 24. The drugs and the radiation did their job. Most peoples white count is between 5,000 and 8,000. So now it's time to wait and watch for the counts to start coming up. Well, three days after the bone marrow transplant, Rocky felt sick and they needed to find out what was wrong. They did more tests including a Bronch in which they insert a tube down your throat to look inside the lungs. The result of that was RSV Pneumonia with a 105.8 degree temperature. RSV is only contracted by babies and bone marrow patients with no immune system. It is also very contagious to this group. So of course Rocky happened to be the first person in this hospital to get RSV. The place went 'up for grabs' trying to figure out how to treat him and not to endanger other BMT patients.

Well, the solution was a plastic tent over Rocky's bed with its own filtration system, which had to be changed every two hours. He had to lay under the tent with an oxygen mask while drugs were taking affect for 18 out of 24 hours. You wouldn't believe what went through my mind as I sat and watched, wearing a mask that made me look as if I had just gotten out of a bomber plane. They asked me to please leave the room when he was sleeping, so I would not be exposed to the drugs; the side effects were still unknown. As I watched the nurses come in, dressed in full gowns, masks, and gloves (some wouldn't even enter), I would sometimes say out loud, "Oh dear God, please take care of my Rocky." On the 10th day his count started to come up...later the doctors said without the count kicking in like that, we would have lost him. Thank you again Lord, for the families and churches who prayed for us in our time of need. Rocky had some rough times, as I remember the milestones. Like the first day he didn't throw up a spoonful of Jell-O or pudding, or the day of his first bite of food that stayed down for more than 10 minutes. I remember him being able to take a shower standing up on his own, being able to talk on the phone, and his first pass out of the hospital for a couple of hours; the day we went home together, 59 days later, PRAISE GOD.

Because of low counts and being on an IV, the environment had to be as sterile as possible. I had the house painted, and we bought new carpeting and furniture. We had to get rid of the dog, the cat, the parrot, and all of the plants. We have great friends that took them all for one year. Then when you think you can come home and start trying to have a normal life, you realize things don't happen that way; the road is long. We had home care nurses for a week until they taught me how to give Rocky his IV meds. One drug would give him tremors where he would shake uncontrollably. I would give him an IV flush and then a drug to make him sleep so he wouldn't get the tremors. Then his other medication would be administered. It was one of the most scary things, but you do what you have to do. Each day we would look for improvement. We took three trips to the doctor's office per week. Just when you would get used to one routine, they would change it. Giving Rocky his meds was a full time job. During his cat naps I would clean, wash clothes, cook, and mow the lawn...then it was finally bedtime. Only guess who doesn't sleep and has to get up 4 or 5 times a night? The hospital was hard, but this is what you would call doubly hard. There were no nurses around to ask me how I am, or to tell me that we're here for you if you need something. Now I was on a time schedule to play all of the roles; the homemaker, a wife, and of course a nurse. There were nights I was so physically exhausted that I couldn't even cry, but then there were lots of days that I did. One side of most of us says, "We can do it." When someone asks me what they can do to help, I say, "Nothing, just pray." I guess sometimes, you really don't know what you need. This is when you are thankful for friends that just come in and take charge. I thank the Lord for them, they just always seem to show up when they are needed.

Well, things do get better each day, and as I look back over all we have been through, I know the Lord is good. At this time, Rocky is back to work full time at his job for Pearl Baths Inc., covering 7 states now. He loves his job. He also speaks out against steroids when he can. But as for ever having a normal life...never. We take each day and thank God for Rocky's extension in life. Some of us never get a second chance. All I can say is that his mission isn't accomplished yet. People will ask Rocky how he gets through each day, and he'll quote Philippians 4:13 from his Bible, "I can do all things through Christ, which strengthens me."

WE LOVE YOU ALL

These precious words told by Rocky's wife Trudy were straight from the heart. The true facts from this incredible story were written with dignity. Nobody could ever imagine the difficulties this couple went through unless they have experienced a similar situation themselves. Trudy deserves loads of credit for her pain and sufferings in getting through all of that.

The man who deserves credit for using every ounce of his willpower just to survive is the one and only Mr. Norman "Rocky" Rauch.

And saving the best for last, as Trudy pointed out in her story, we all should praise the Lord each and every day of our lives. Amen.

CHAPTER 11
THE COMMITMENT OF A LIFETIME

Fifty-nine days was an unusual amount of time for a bone marrow transplant victim to be in the hospital; most of them were out in less than half that amount of time. Rocky had been an athlete all of his life, and he knew all the odds of winning championships. You have a 50 percent chance; you either win or you lose.

One morning during his visit with the medical world, Rocky's brain was actually functioning correctly by the grace of God. He had been filled with drugs and powerful radiation treatments beyond belief. "For the first time in my life, I realize one thing," whispered Rocky to anyone who was nearby. "I am going to be a winner both ways. If I live, I can be useful and resourceful. I can be an extension for Christ. And if I die, I go home to be with him because I already have made that commitment."

Paul Molitor visited Rocky a number of times during his unforgettable stay in the hospital. This athlete became a very personal and special friend of Rocky's. The superstar would go out and speak to people on behalf of the Fellowship of Christian Athletes. When Paul would show up at the hospital, all the nurses would go stir crazy and want to meet him and get his autograph. One day Rocky's head doctor, Dr. Horowitz, asked Paul if he could go down to the floor below Rocky's and talk to a young boy who had terminal cancer. So Paul Molitor of the Milwaukee Brewers walked into this kid's room unannounced. The boy recognized Paul right away and asked, "Paul Molitor, what are you doing here?" The teenager was never told that he only had one week left on God's green earth. Trudy was also in the boy's room with Paul, who glanced over at her with a tear in his eye.

Being somewhat of an emotional person, Paul spoke to the young lad, "We'll be praying with you, son, that hopefully you will be all right." The boy got to meet the celebrity of his dreams before he passed away ten days later.

Paul would even call Trudy when he was on the road to inquire about Rocky's condition, and he always wanted to know how she was holding up. That's just the kind of a giving athlete that he was.

The leader of the Fellowship of Christian Athletes talked to Trudy just before Rocky's birthday and asked, "What movie star celebrity or sports figure would Rocky want to invite to his birthday party?"

"That's an easy one," snickered Trudy. "Of course Rocky would want Sylvester Stallone to show up here at the hospital for his birthday."

"What would be his second choice?" asked Dean, the leader. "This other Rocky guy might just be a little hard to get a hold of."

"Then I would have to say Mike Ditka," answered Trudy.

Four days later, Dean called Trudy and said, "I have some good news and some bad news. The coach of the Chicago Bears, Iron Mike, has another engagement and won't be able to come to the hospital. But the good news is that he has prepared a video tape of himself that we will set up for Rocky to watch on his birthday."

Tears of joy were rolling down Rocky's cheeks as he watched that video tape of Mike Ditka talking to him. Rocky and his brother Charlie watched some of the Chicago Bears games together before he was admitted to the hospital. Rocky was even mistaken for Iron Mike a couple of times because both had the same facial features, and both had the physiques of an iron bridge.

Despite having spent fifty-nine days in the hospital as a bone marrow transplant recipient, Rocky still had many complications as an outpatient for around six months. Most companies would only carry you for maybe thirty days' worth of disability compensation, but because the owner of Pearl Baths was so compassionate, Rocky was sent commission checks while he was in the hospital. Trudy had written, from her heart, a piece called "Rocky's Road" (printed in the previous chapter), and sent it to Pearl, who in return sent a copy to every one of Rocky's customers.

Rocky was off to a slow start after being released from the hospital on March 29, 1990. The road was long and treacherous as he tried to get back to the grindstone. He still had his customer representative job, the work that he loved dearly. The clientele that he had built up through the years thought of him as a brother and a hero.

While back out in the workforce, Rocky was still required to show up at his clinic three times a week for routine checkups. One day he noticed a giant poster at the clinic on the bulletin board. It was all about the Transplant Olympic Games that were to take place toward the end of the summer. Rocky inquired about this competition and received a packet in the mail. The Transplant Games were to consist of such events as bicycling, golfing, a baseball throw, badminton, ping pong, tennis, 5K and 10K races, 440 and 880 relay races, shot put, and more. When Rocky first read about this event, he wasn't strong enough to tear his cereal box in half to discard of it. Trudy had to do that for him. But he had never been a quitter in his life, and he had big ideas about getting his strength back up to enter the shot put competition.

When he tried lifting the Olympic-size sixteen-pound shot put, he could hardly get it up to his waist with both hands. Rocky was able to put that sixteen-pound shot a mile in his earlier days, just for the fun of it.

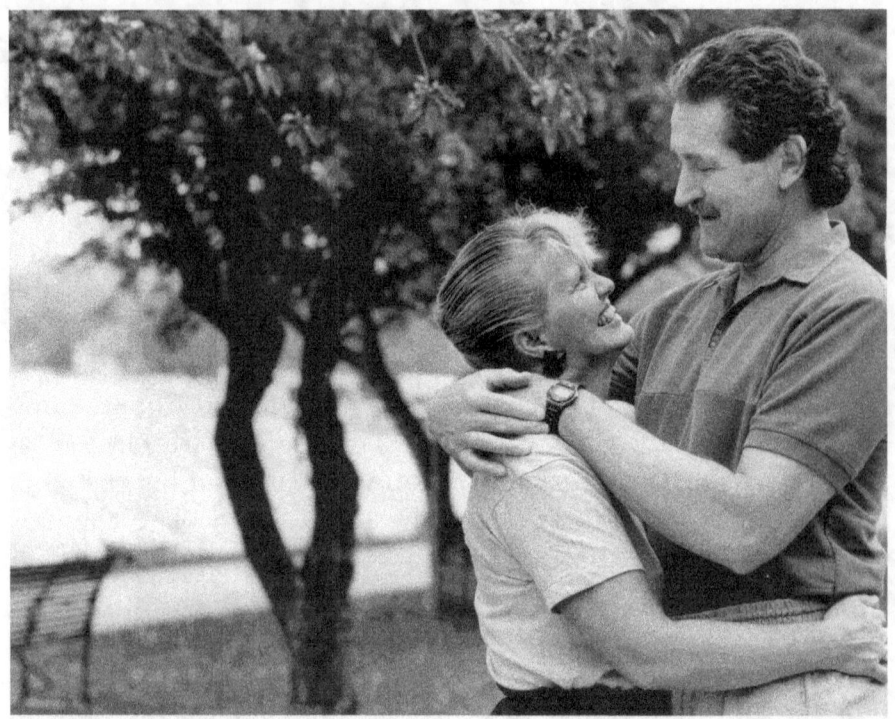

Wife Trudy has "been there"
for Rocky every step of the
way — caring for him when
he was ill, now training with
him and cheering him on toward his new goals

There were approximately nine weeks to train before the Pur-
due Transplant Olympic Games. The closest location for Norm to
start his training was the high school yard, about half a mile from
his house. Trudy would wake up with her husband every morning
at five o'clock and go over to the field to help him to get ready for
the games. On weekends she would bring the video camera out to
the field to tape her husband in action. This way he could play the
tapes back to determine what he might be doing wrong. Rocky was
still on different types of medication. It was not easy to train hard,
against the medication, to build his strength back. Trudy was out
there almost every day to practice with him and support him.

A group of sponsors from Wisconsin put on big fundraisers while
the team of Wisconsin transplant athletes was in training. Some of the

sponsors raised over $2,500 for each transplant trainee to be able to participate in the Transplant Games. Just before this huge self-endurance competition, Rocky and Trudy drove to Purdue University in Indiana to meet for something that he had strived hard all his life to do: win! Rocky always had a hard time dealing with anything other than first place. He always gave everything he had to every competition he was involved in.

BONE MARROW TRANSPLANTS *A New*

Weapon Against Cancer

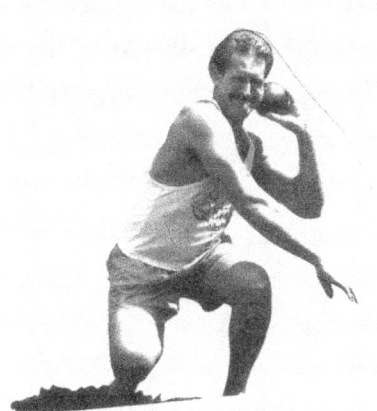

"THE ROCK IS BACK"

All his life, Rocky had dreamed about competing in the Olympic Games. Due to injuries in the past, his dreams had never come true, but now he was given a chance to compete against a heart transplant recipient from New York in the Transplant Olympics.

On his attempt, the athlete from New York tripped on the toe-block that was attached to the seven-foot shot put ring and fouled. He landed on his wrist and sprained it. The New Yorker made one more attempt but couldn't get a throw in because of the wrist injury. There were only two competitors in this age group, so all Rocky had to do for the gold was to make one put of the shot count. The hard, long hours of practicing paid off for the big man. Three attempts were performed, and twenty-two feet, ten inches was his best shot. Rocky had finally fulfilled his dream. He had won the GOLD METAL!

In the ceremony after all of the events took place, Rocky (while popping buttons off his shirt) went up to receive his most valuable prize. Karl Lewis presented Rocky with his medal by putting it around his neck.

In the Olympic Games of 1988, Karl was the athlete who competed for a gold medal against Den Johnsen, who was eventually disqualified for steroid use.

As Karl did the honors, Rocky just had to put his two cents in and say a few words to him. "You and I have something in common. You received your gold medal because of your competitor being on steroids. You are presenting me with a gold medal because I used steroids, which caused me to have a transplant after getting cancer."

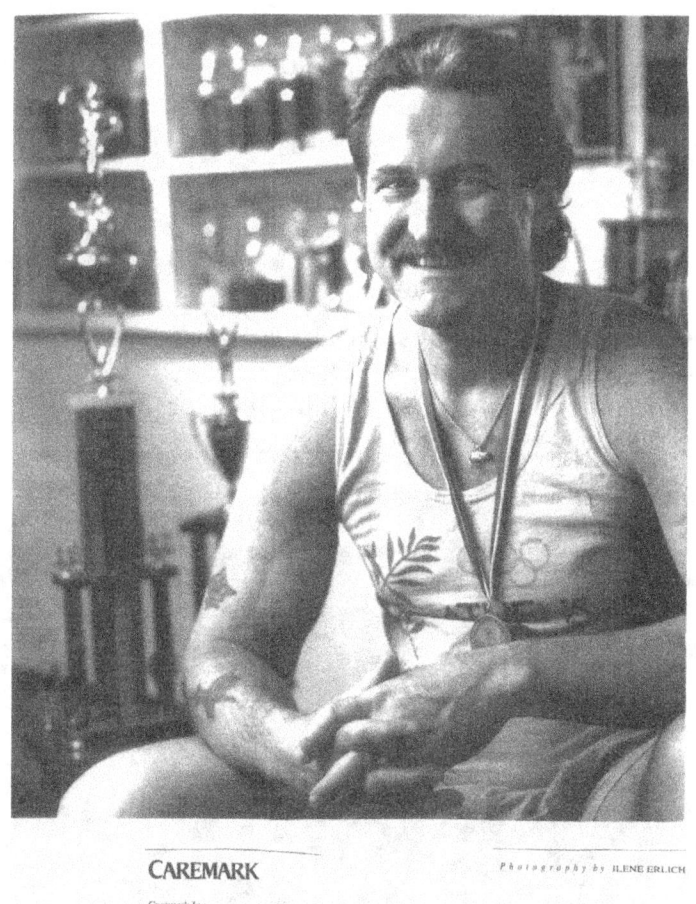

CAREMARK

Photography by ILENE ERLICH

Caremark Inc.
Affiliate Baxter Healthcare Corporation
455 Knightsbridge Parkway

Rocky treasured this prestigious medal of honor because he earned this title by being drug-free...or was he? Some of the transplant athletes jokingly said, "We don't use steroids, but do you think that they will drug test us anyway?" But actually, some of them did use prescribed steroids. Rocky himself was on a prescribed medication for catabolic steroids.

This achievement of taking part in the Transplant Games was only the beginning. After that accomplishment, Rocky found out about the World Transplant games that were to take place in Budapest, Hungary. For this worldwide competition, Rocky and Trudy would have to raise their own funding in excess of $5,000 just to get there for Rocky to participate. They did not know where they were going to get their hands on $5,000, but since Rocky had his heart set on going, he acquired the necessary forms to fill out and the approval from his doctor. As he was filling out one of the forms, Rocky did not see bone marrow transplant listed, so he wrote it in himself.

With the help and support from Channel 6 TV and Dean from the Fellowship of Christian Athletes, they were able to put a huge fundraiser together. A couple of Green Bay football players and a professional basketball player from North Carolina became involved. They called themselves the All-Star Team to help Rocky achieve another one of his goals. Large posters were set up that read, "Send Rocky to Budapest!"

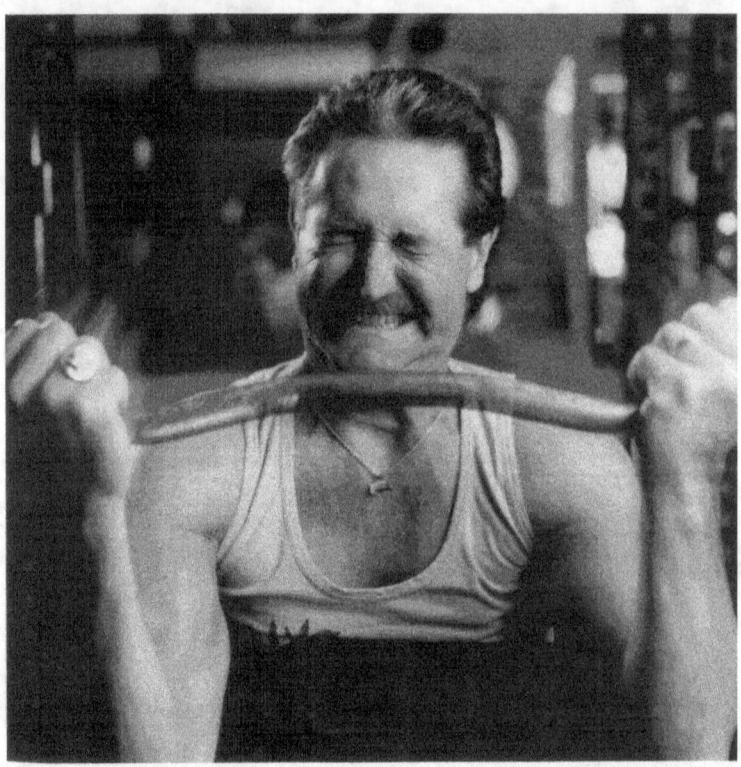

Former "Mr. America" Rocky Rauch now pumps iron with the same determination and intensity that helped him win his battle over cancer.

The All-Star Team participated in a fundraiser basketball game that was held in Lake Geneva at the Badger High School. The mayor and some of the town dignitaries, like the chief of police and fire chief, put together the opposing team. Paul Molitor and the triple-threat Brewer athletes donated numerous autographed items to be auctioned off. Rocky gave his presentation at half time. This major event was publicized through the distribution of many posters and local radio station broadcasts.

The special thing about this fundraiser was that many of the local taxpayers gave their support to put it on. Pizza Hut donated twenty or more pizzas, and McDonald's threw in free soda for all of the athletes and spectators to enjoy after the game. It seemed like the entire community was pitching in to raise the $5,000 that Rocky and his wife needed to go to Budapest to fulfill Rocky's dream.

Two weeks before take-off, a gal from a local clothing store printed ROCKY and TRUDY on bright red sweatshirts (with the Badger emblem) for the couple to wear in Budapest. At the city council meeting, the mayor gave Rocky the Lake Geneva flag to display over there. Eighty-two people who were representing the United States, along with some spouses and friends, flew from Milwaukee, Wisconsin, to New York. From New York, they all were transported to Zurich, Switzerland, and then to the final destination: Budapest.

Upon arrival, the United States citizens were chauffeured to their motel. It was more like army barracks with pull-chain toilets and strange-looking cots to sleep on. Rocky had trained very hard back in the States for the fifty-meter breaststroke and the fifty-meter freestyle swimming competitions and of course the shot put event. His strength was gradually coming back, and he felt pumped and ready more than ever to win the priceless World Transplant gold medal.

The first night in Budapest, one of the team leaders walked up to Rocky and said, "I have some bad news for you, sir. The International Committee just met, and they concluded that you are ineligible. You cannot compete."

What a letdown for the man who wanted to be the best at whatever he did in life! "I've been working hard for a year now and my enthusiasm is built up, and now that I'm finally here, you're telling me that I can't compete?" replied Rocky. "I legally sent in my entry forms, and they accepted my money. What kind of idiots are running this show anyway?" Trudy, Rocky, and their close friends were just devastated by this unbelievable news. Rocky finished his second Hungarian beer and ventured outside on his own. The beer helped to put his state of mind into rare form.

The guy who had delivered the devastating news followed Rocky outside and spoke, "I'm sorry about the news, Rocky, so if you want to relieve some anxiety by throwing that beer bottle, I'll understand."

"You don't understand," interrupted Rocky. "You don't understand anything. I went through an out-of-the-ordinary transplant, you might say, and then all of my friends and people I don't even know gave up their valuable time to put on a fundraiser for me to get over here. My community supported me 100 percent, and now you want me to go back home and tell them that I was disqualified because I was ineligible. How stupid is that?"

"Well, I'm really sorry," explained the team leader.

"You'd better go back in there and tell them that I'm not taking this news very lightly," demanded Rocky. "Furthermore, I'll go in there and give them a piece of my mind. How many bone marrow transplant people are here anyway? Are we that big of a threat?" There were over 750 athletes who qualified to be in the World Transplant Games from thirty-one different countries. "This is a huge affair, and I worked very hard to get here."

"Let me see what I can do," replied the team leader.

Rocky and Trudy went back to their room. She was very upset with this entire ordeal, and he felt more rejected now than he ever had in his lifetime. Soon after they were conversing with each other, the telephone rang. "I have some good news for you and also some not-so-good news," explained the leader.

"What is this, one of those good news/bad news jokes?" asked Rocky.

"Well, no. The good news is that they're going to let you compete, but you are not going to be able to compete for a medal," replied the team leader.

"No big deal," answered Rocky.

"So what is your answer, then? Are you going to compete?"

"What do you think I'm going to do?" interrupted Rocky, slightly raising his tone of voice. "I came all the way over here for the challenge to win, and that's what I'm going to do. Forget your precious medals!" Not overjoyed with his first visit to this foreign country, Rocky went into the lobby and started to mingle with some of his friends. The word about what was happening was spreading like wildfire.

One of the athletes yelled out, "This is preposterous! They can't do this to a man who came a long way through the healing process by the grace of God."

Another friend of Rocky's spoke up, "We might just have to have a little discussion here about boycotting the games. If they don't let you compete for a medal, then we shouldn't compete either."

Rocky had to state his feelings on this touchy subject. "You guys have worked very hard to get here, just like I have. I know this means a lot to all of us. But you don't need to jeopardize your athletic competition for me. Great Britain athletes have won this a lot in the past, and I believe there are more spokesmen on the International Committee from Great Britain than anywhere else. I just think that this is a big rip off. So all I'm saying is let's get out there and beat the crap out of the British!"

Let the games begin. The fifty-meter freestyle swimming event took place, and Rocky acquired the third-best time for his team. They wanted to use him at the end of the competition for the relay race until someone remembered that he was not eligible for a medal, which meant that the team would not be eligible either. The team competed in the freestyle relay race without Rocky and won, but it was a crying shame that Rocky was not able to take part in that event.

It was now time for the shot put event that Rocky trained extra hard for. His best put of the shot was twenty-nine feet, eight inches. This guaranteed him third place in the preliminaries. So the American representative was now eligible to compete in the finals…or so he was told at the beginning of the World Transplant Games. The German team was in first place, the Norwegians were in second, Rocky was in third, representing the United States, and France was in fourth. When the list of names came up with the eight team finalists, Rocky's name was not called. He didn't waste any time in going straight up to present his argument with one of the committee members.

"What the devil is going on here?" asked Rocky. "I'm supposed to be in the finals."

"You're not eligible to win a medal," replied the committee member.

"Now wait a minute here," shouted Rocky. "You said that I could compete, and to me that means until the very end." The International Committee members met once again to make a decision pertaining to this special issue. They took a vote, and the majority ruled to let Rocky proceed in the shot put competition all the way through the grand finale. The committee informed Rocky from the beginning to keep this matter hush-hush so that the other teams would not be disrupted in any way or form. Rocky respected their decision, didn't make much of a scene, and didn't complain except to tell some of his friends that he was very disappointed. So the word about Rocky's issue of not being able to win a medal was pretty much limited to the American teammates.

The old Rocky would have had this matter broadcast around the world by now, but the new and improved Rocky's thought process took him back to the beginning ceremonies. "It was quite an honor to be selected by my teammates to carry the American flag past the reviewing stand of judges. There were thirty-one different flags waving by with their national anthems playing at that precise moment. I didn't hold any tears back, as I thought, 'What an honor it is to be here, representing my great country.' I will never forget this moment in time."

The day of the finals, Rocky tossed the shot put a total distance of twenty-nine feet, ten inches, which allowed him to hold onto third place. At that point Trudy was there encouraging him, taking numerous photographs, and just cheering her husband on to victory. But as time went on that day, she felt that it was very wrong for her husband not to be rewarded for his accomplishments.

And just think about what she had accomplished! If Trudy hadn't been there for Rocky during those fifty-nine days in the hospital and then playing nurse, housewife, chief cook and bottle washer, and caretaker, would he have survived? During the award ceremony, Trudy disappeared. She decided to drift off and do something for herself; a nearby spa and shopping mall looked pretty inviting.

The athlete from France was called up to receive the bronze medal. He could not believe what he was hearing. It was difficult for Rocky to watch this French guy get up on the platform when he knew that he had earned the medal, but he just nonchalantly shook his head, turned around, and was just about ready to go look for his wife.

Right there in his face was the entire United States team.

"You can't leave yet, Mr. Rauch," stated one of Rocky's teammates. "We need the same guy who carried our stars and stripes into this festival to also lead us out to go back home as champions!"

"Well, I don't know if I really deserve to do that," replied Rocky. "Let someone else have the glory."

"We want you to carry our flag, Mr. Rauch," demanded his teammates in unison.

Rocky did the job that was requested of him for the closing ceremonies, and then it was finally time to leave the country and go back home. When they arrived back in Zurich, Switzerland, for the layover, Trudy was called up to the front of the group. She was met by their team leader. Then Curt, a kidney transplant recipient from Madison, Wisconsin, signaled for Rocky to come up to the head of the class. Curt was a great athlete, even before his transplant, and he had won about half a dozen medals at the World Games.

"I want you to have this medal in remembrance of the Games," said Curt with open arms.

"Wow!" exclaimed Rocky. "But I can't accept this. You won it fair and square."

Rocky was eventually presented with the bronze medal (hung around his neck by Trudy), from Wynn, an extraordinary swimmer. "This is for you, my man," said Wynn. "All of us standing right here believe that you are worthy of this bronze medal more than anyone else in the universe. Am I right, guys?"

The team cheered in reply.

CHAPTER 12
THE REAL ROCKY, WITHOUT
THE ATTITUDE

Back near Lake Geneva, there was no motorcade to pick up Rocky and his wife at the airport. There was not even a parade scheduled in Rocky's honor to float down Lake Geneva Boulevard on Sunday afternoon. Actually, only a couple of their neighbors had heard what took place over in Budapest. When people would ask how well he did over there, Rocky would answer, "I received the bronze medal in the shot put competition."

Rocky just had to find out who the President of the International Transplant Committee was, and why "bone marrow transplant recipient" was not listed on the World Games application form. By doing some research and making a few telephone calls, Rocky found out that the president was a doctor from Great Britain. He came up with the idea of putting a petition together. If he could get hundreds or maybe even one thousand signatures, then just maybe Rocky could pull this off in favor of the bone marrow transplant recipients. "Where there's a will, there's a way" had always been Rocky's philosophy.

Although he has often tried to help people, Norman was starting to see life through a different set of spectacles. He had another perspective on life, a change of the heart and attitude, you could say. He not only wanted to do some good for people but also wanted to be closer to his family and serve our great Lord in a better fashion. Rocky was actually starting to realize that the Lord doesn't want us to always request favors of him. The message was being sent to Rocky to focus more on praying about learning more about Jesus Christ through worship and his teachings.

Thus far, bone marrow transplant athletes had been able to compete in the United States Games but not in the World Games. In the next year, Rocky was able to put together a petition with over 2,000 names. A letter was also written by his doctor explaining exactly what a bone marrow transplant consisted of. The Transplant Committee proclaimed that this type of procedure did not involve organs and was not life-threatening. After what Rocky went through, he could not believe that people in the medical world could ever make a statement like that.

In 1992, Rocky took his petition and entered the shot put event in the United States Games in Los Angeles. He was focused more on getting his medical letter and petition recognized. His heart wasn't in the competition like it had been in Budapest. He still had a sore spot because of what happened over there. But Rocky wanted to see his familiar comrades doing what they do best.

Rocky would never forget when he asked a lady who had had a kidney transplant years ago to sign his petition. He was very offended when she said, "Well, you don't have to take anti-rejection drugs and be on a tight schedule for the rest of your life. If they're going to let people like you in, they might as well let cornea transplant recipients into the World Games." She said that she would not sign the petition.

In Vancouver in 1993, this issue was voted on, and the decision was made to allow bone marrow transplant recipients to compete in the World Games. Rocky had accomplished another one of his goals: to help part of mankind to reach theirs.

Thinking back to when he was married to his first wife, Rocky felt that he had caused a lot of his own problems through his dedication to his sport. He also believed that he could have excelled at his job if he would have given more effort, although some people gave him more praise than he actually took credit for. In his prime, Rocky's gym life was more important to him than his family. It was like working two jobs: his work to make a living and working out to master the opportunity to be an Olympic champion.

His oldest daughter Sally told her father that he was never there for her and some mental scars were left for her to ponder upon from time to time. Every kid needs a father. Rocky's daughters were deprived of their father's comfort every day, at a very early stage in their lives. After the divorce, he could only be with them one or two weekends out of the month.

Sometimes tables turn as we go through life. Rocky's younger brother was always envious of him because of all his glory and awards, but when Rocky thought about how successful his brother was in the business world and that he could still devote most of his off-time to his three sons, he felt a sense of jealousy.

Having a different perspective on life, Rocky realized that he had devoted more time to his sport than to his first three wives— maybe not at first, but eventually he would get bored and spend less time at home. He remembered getting the ultimatum from his third wife before the big Wisconsin competition: he could not compete, or she would leave him. When his father had been rather ill before his greatest achievement, the Mr. America contest, he remembered thinking that it would be a shame if his father died and he couldn't compete.

Rocky looked back at all these different situations and realized that maybe he did not have his priorities in order. He should have been more concerned about other people than himself.

Rocky had begun to understand that faith should be number one on everyone's priority list. He believed that the association with God kept him stable. This used to be fourth on his list.

Your family should come second. A father needs to spend a great deal of time with his kids. They need as much attention as they can get, especially when they are going through school. You should be there for their band concerts, graduation ceremonies, and theatrical plays.

Next in line would be your profession, a way to earn money to support your family, but you do not need to make that your whole life either.

You should always put yourself last. Don't put yourself down; just don't let your ego take over when other people are present. Most people don't appreciate hearing you brag about yourself.

When Rocky got out of the hospital after the transplant, his life took a 180-degree turn. His priorities were just the opposite of what they used to be when he was trying to win every competition in sight. We are all creatures of habit, and sometimes it's very difficult to break old habits. Most people are stuck in the same pattern day in, day out. Rocky became more flexible than he had ever been in his life. It took a good woman, his fourth wife, to put him in line.

Most teenage boys take everything for granted. That's the way Norman Rauch was growing up. He began speaking to kids in high schools who had no fear of death whatsoever. They didn't understand it, so why should they think about it? It was like they only thought of older people dying. "I'm invincible! Nothing can happen to me!"

When Rocky was around 40 years of age, he didn't see anyone keeling over from steroid use. He knew it was wrong, and he knew it could be life-threatening, but he still didn't have a fear of death at that time. It takes someone like a professional doctor saying, "You have cancer. Your life is on the line. You could die," before you experience the rude awakening.

Rocky sometimes wondered if older people who had cancer thought, "Well, I've lived my life. So what if I die?" Maybe some people gave up at that age. But wouldn't it be nice if they could be treated so they could live another twenty years of a fruitful life with their grandkids? God didn't put us on this earth to give up at anything. He put us on this land to make the best of our lives.

There were many arguments that Rocky had with his ex-wives about the past. He would constantly bring up past experiences to throw in their faces. His new philosophy was much different: the past is gone, and you can never bring it back, so don't even worry about it. It is wise to cherish the good memories and try to forget about the bad ones. Just live one day at a time. Try to have a great experience with Jesus Christ every day.

Weightlifting was now behind Rocky. If he worked out for his health, that was fine. If he didn't, so what? Some people try to run three miles a day for exercise and if for some reason they can't fit that into their schedule, it throws them off-kilter. This is the way Rocky used to be with his bodybuilding. But now he felt that there was always tomorrow for your hobbies. Family comes before hobbies, and also one must strive hard at his job to support the family.

Things are too easy today in life, Rocky would say from time to time. So many people are on welfare, which is too easy to collect. He thought that you should be supportive in the best possible way: by self-endurance and earning every possible Lincoln-head yourself. Some people out there purposely commit crimes to go to jail, where, under certain circumstances it's like being at a health club. You have gyms, and you get fed your three square meals a day. Sure, you are locked up, but some maniacs enjoy this routine. It's a life of no responsibility. In society today, the leaders make it too easy and too comfortable for people to do nothing. Rocky's father Henry always told him that there were too many do-nothings out there, people who thought you owed them everything but did not want to return the favor.

The new and improved Rocky was very pleased with his new lifestyle. When he walked into a crowd of people, he didn't want them to look at him like he was Mr. Hot Shot. Ego-tripping was not his specialty anymore, although he was proud of what he did. When he was involved with speaking to kids about steroid abuse, he wasn't doing it for the recognition. He just wanted to reach out to every kid he could get his hands on and tell them how bad it is for them. Out of a thousand kids, if one decided that steroids were harmful, then Rocky felt that he had accomplished his goal for that day. He didn't worry about what was going to happen the next day anymore.

Rocky kept track of how many days it had been since his transplant. This is what he called his second chance at life, the extension that God gave him. The doctors said that after being in remission for five years, a cancer victim should be almost all the way out of the woods.

Rocky recalled an experience from when he was in his first year with Pearl Bath. On his way to Wausau, Wisconsin, he thought about the meeting with his distributor and knew he had to call on his account. He felt that he should go buy himself a new pair of dress shoes to upgrade his appearance, so he walked into this Floor Shine shoe store when he arrived in town. He just wanted something simple: a pair of loafers with tassels on the top front of the shoes. Rocky found a pair of shoes that he liked and asked the saleswoman if he could wear them out of the store. She replied, "Certainly you may, sir, and could I also interest you in a dog?"

"I thought this was a shoe store, not a pet store," snickered Rocky.

"Actually, my boyfriend and I have a miniature poodle," explained the salesgirl. "My boyfriend works long hours as a car salesman, and I'm here late a lot, so we have to leave our puppy locked in the bathroom. He is only eight weeks old and is the cutest little guy you'd ever want to lay your eyes on. I guess he doesn't fit into our lifestyle. Would you want to give him a good home?"

"Well, I don't know," answered Rocky. "I just can't take a dog without talking to my wife first. I'll tell you what. I'll be back either tomorrow or the next day to let you know what we decide, all right?" So Rocky called Trudy about this little mongrel, and she said she'd like to see him. Rocky called that salesgirl back and was told to meet at their house the next night.

When he walked into their house, there was a small cage set up by the front door with two dog bowls, a leash, and doggy snacks nearby. All of a sudden this small creature scampered out of the bathroom and gave a mighty big roar for its size.

"We call him Handsome," said the girl. The little thing looked cute, curly, and cuddly. He was all black with a tan beard, four tan paws, and a tan chest.

Rocky's first impulse was to say, "How you doing, little old man?" He picked him up, and the dog fit comfortably into the palm of his hand. Little Handsome started to lick Norman's wrist. This was the cutest little thing that he had ever seen. The big man fell in love with the "little old man" right off the bat.

The little poodle sat in Rocky's lap (not wearing a seatbelt), all the way back home that evening. When Trudy saw the little guy curled up in her husband's huge arm entering the front foyer, she just totally fell in love with this precious animal. They decided to think of a better name for him immediately, something that would welcome him into the household. A Siamese cat with the sophisticated name of Rambo had already occupied this residency for some time.

Rocky wanted to call the little puppy Arnold, after the muscle-bound man who eventually became the governor of California. Trudy was definitely all right with the name. Now this lucky couple had a couple of pets: a lap dog named Arnold, and Rambo the Siamese cat. I wonder which one will be the luckiest to get there first to empty the tuna cans. You never know when man's best friend might get catlike symptoms. When their hair stands on end, their tails go straight up, and they do a 360-degree spin in midair—and can still land on their feet after jumping off the living room chandelier—then you'll know for sure.

THE TALE OF TWO KEYS
(FOR ROCKY'S TWO CITIES)

What could be a better gift of honor than to receive a golden key to your own city? The Mayor of Lake Geneva, Wisconsin, presented Norman Henry Rauch with this cherished token that he would always be grateful for. A proclamation was also received because of Rocky's outlandish efforts to bring former Milwaukee Brewer Paul Molitor into the city to raise funds for baseball diamonds. Showing their appreciation for the ex-Brewer Mr. Igniter coming around, the rotary club named one of the many baseball fields The Paul Molitor Baseball Diamond in his honor.

Sports
Lake Geneva Regional News

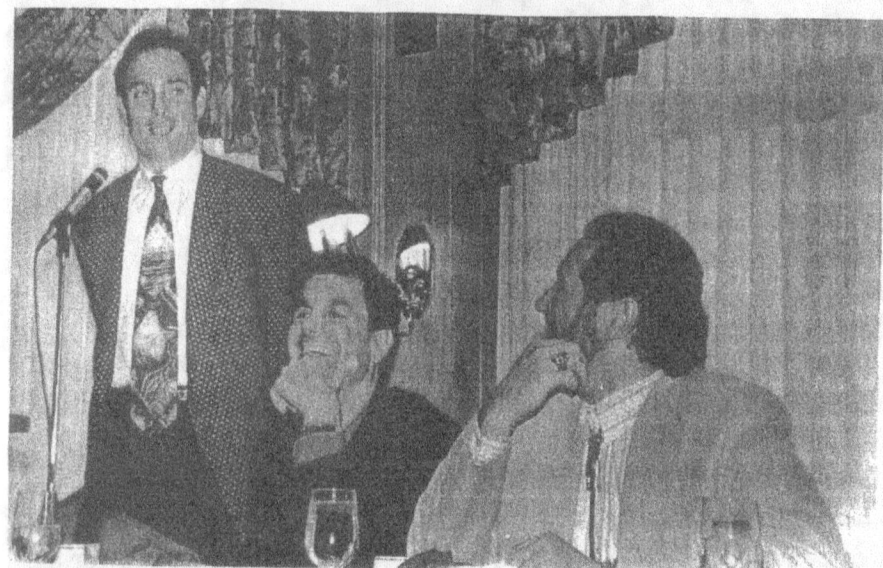

MILWAUKEE BREWERS designated hitter/first baseman Paul Molitor reflected on some of the humorous moments of the past season while speaking at a Lake Geneva Rotary Club luncheon to benefit the fields at Veterans Memorial Park. Laughing at one of Molitor's anecdotes are WITI Milwaukee channel 6 Sports Director Tom Pipines (middle) and Norman "Rocky" Rauch of Lake Geneva. Rauch, a bronze medalist at the 1991 World Transplant Games in Budapest, Hungary, was instrumental in attracting Molitor and Pipines for the fund raiser. The three men are good friends and members of the Fellowship of Christian Athletes. Regional News Photo

Molitor Benefit Raises Funds for Veterans Park

The man with a thousand stories to tell also received the key to his hometown where he grew up: Allentown, Pennsylvania. When Rocky went back home after thirty-one years, the mayor proclaimed it Rocky Rauch Day. He was the fourth person in history to be honored with this priceless possession. The three previous keys went out to two former presidents and a congressman.

Rocky made it an obligation to sit in at the DARE graduation ceremony in Fond du Lac County, which was strictly organized by the sheriff's department.

There's not much more that you can say about this giant of a man, except that God Almighty wanted him to continue on with his purpose in life: to explain to kids what this earth's stepping stone is all about before they're granted the key to Heaven's gate.

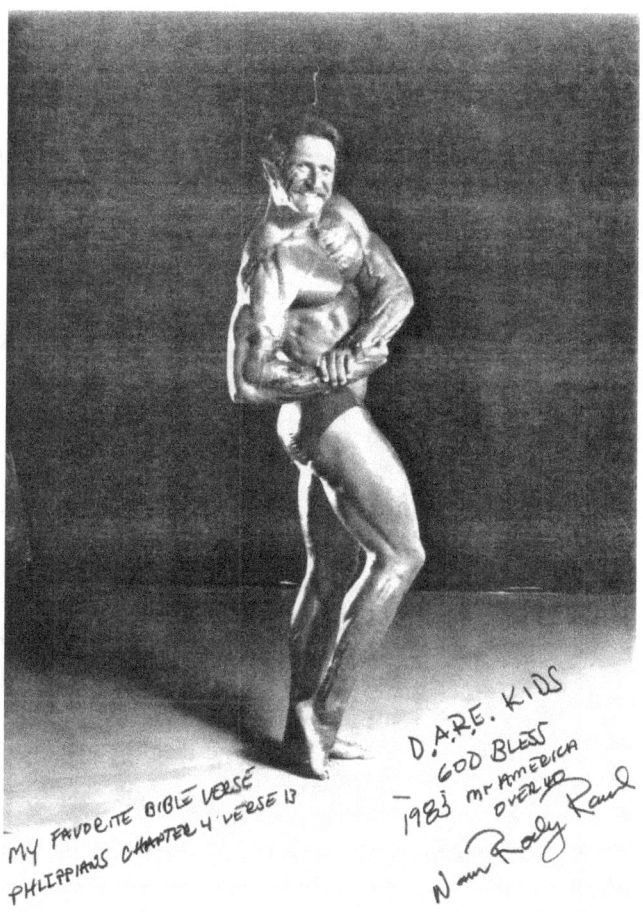

MY FAVORITE BIBLE VERSE
PHILIPPIANS CHAPTER 4 VERSE 13

D.A.R.E. KIDS
GOD BLESS
1983 MR AMERICA
OVER 40
Nown Rudy Raul

ROCKY'S RIDE IS NOT OVER
Epilogue

This giant of a man was greatly inspired by two men of the cloth in the twenty-first century. These two great names will probably go down in history someday, especially in Jesus Christ's book. The first is a faithful man with more spunk in his nature than a Wisconsin gray squirrel crossing in your pathway. The following story is the testimony that was presented by Pastor Reggie at Trinity Lutheran Church (TLC), on August 15, 2004, when Rocky was in the front pew:

I was on my way to give my presentation to the congregation at a church in Racine, Wisconsin. Getting slightly disoriented, I somehow got off the beaten path and ended up in Kenosha. My cell phone was at hand, so I dialed a number for better directions. I realized at the moment that police officers do not like for you to drive with only one hand on the steering wheel. So as I looked out of my rearview and side view mirrors, I reached with my other hand to make sure my collar was in place. I guess at that particular moment, the car was operating by itself. Well, it looks like I have everything under control now, or do I?

When I arrived into the parking lot at the church, I felt that something was not quite right. It was the middle of January, and the asphalt was covered with frozen snow. I remember having a difficult time parking my vehicle…and not because there were no vacant parking spaces. Finally coming to a standstill, which seemed like an eternity, I was not able to remove myself from the driver's seat. All of a sudden my peripheral vision was lost. Then my frontal vision was narrowed down to the size of a beach ball. Everything else on both sides of my cheeks were dark, darker than my own skin. Then my depleting brainwaves relayed a message to my left arm, "Please release the door handle and open the darn door." My arm did not respond. It was totally numb. Then all of a sudden my frontal vision was reduced to the size of a quarter. This all took place in a matter of moments. The only thing that I could possibly think about was to cry to my Almighty Master for help.

"Dear Lord Jesus," I whispered with every last once of energy, "I believe that I'm going to need your help today. I realize that you are always busy, but I truly believe that this might be an essential matter. I wanted to be able to talk to these wonderful folks today at this beautifully-constructed home of yours."

Out of the grace of God, I was able to push open the door and slide out of my vehicle. When I tried to stand, at that very moment I realized how much of a slippery situation this was going to be. "Please, Lord, I'm asking you once again for your help. Don't let me fall. I don't want to be out here when the church lets out. What if one of those fourteen-year-old kids goes out to get the car for his parents?"

Thanks to some very helpful parishioners coming out of the back door early, Pastor Reggie was rescued, although, the Lord Almighty actually saved Pastor Reggie by hanging on to him the entire time. The pastor was sent this message: "I was holding on to you during your time of need. You must stay on this glorious earth for another mission."

Sitting up front near the limelight, Rocky was feeling a bit emotional and was intrigued by Pastor Reggie's message. He felt that he still had a mission in life: to get through to his kids about the effects of steroids.

Reggie went on to talk about visiting an elderly lady in the hospital on her death bed:

When I first walked into the room, I didn't know if this 80-pound woman was even still breathing, so I tapped her on the shoulder. All of a sudden she reached up, tugged on my lapels and spoke, "I will never let you go until you pray for me."

Then I said, "Pray for yourself, lady, and please just let loose of me. What would people think if they opened the door to this room right now?"

Well, this sickly-looking woman had more strength than Godzilla. She pulled me down on top of her on the bed. Luckily, nobody entered the hospital room at that particular moment. I eventually prayed with this lady at her request and then sprinted out of the room when she let go of me to sneeze.

Pastor Brian is the second man of the cloth who was always an inspiration for Rocky. He was the head pastor at Trinity Lutheran in Pell Lake, Wisconsin. If you think that Mick Jagger runs around a lot on stage, you should have seen what this down-to-earth (except when he was holding communion) guy was like! Pastor Brian loved to have fun playing with audience members from time to time. This is what the pastor talked about during his sermon on January 2, 2005:

Sometimes people think that if they pray to the Lord Almighty, they should receive a quick response. Well, I'll tell you this is not the way that the Lord works. He has a different perspective. Remember when some of us went out to look at those five acres of land for this new church building to be erected on? We all prayed together about the new location, but then because of all of the red tape involved, that idea fell through. You see, God had another, more powerful idea in mind. He will answer you when the time is right. Months later, we were able to purchase the twenty-three acres that this house of God was eventually built on. It even came equipped with a giant radio antenna and had enough room left over for a huge parking lot.

In the middle of his sermon, Pastor Brian called up all the small children from the pews to come forward. They were going to participate in a taste test. The pastor always had something up his sleeve.

Rocky, you may come up, too, or actually, you can stay seated because the kids are circling around you near the front pew. I want all of you boys and girls to lick your forefinger and stick it into this bowl of white powder I'm passing around. I realize this could be unhealthy and your parents are going to kill me for this. But taste this ingredient and tell me what you think. Go ahead, Rocky. You do the same.

By the expression on your faces, you kids probably think that this stuff is salty and yucky, and you want to poke me in the ribcage. The boys and girls were yelling out, "This stuff tastes awful!" I just want to point out to you guys and parents, that some cooking ingredients taste horrible alone. But if you add a whole bunch of sweet, salty, and sour things together, the final outcome could be Mom's homemade, delicious, mouthwatering apple pie. You kids may go back to your seats now. Rocky, you can stay where you're at.

Folks, you might be struggling with something in your life; it could be an unhappy marriage, not having enough money to pay bills, maybe not being able to make friends. It could be almost anything. Sometimes younger people suffer from teenage depression or peer pressure. Well, you know, all these unhealthy things in our lives could add up to be the not-so-tasty ingredients of the pie. But once that you, the baker, measure and sift through all those ingredients; I assure you that the final product, through the grace of God, will be very tasty in the end.

One night before the holidays, a guy by the name of Dan Mehring came into the church and was excited about sharing a true story with me. A few days before, Dan was at the store with his wife Regina and happened to see a lady walking slowly with long shoelaces dangling off to the sides of her shoes. Most people walking by would have taken that with a grain of salt. A prankster clowning around might have thought, "Have a nice trip. See you in the fall." But this actually bothered Dan, not only because he was a neat freak. He also was afraid that the lady could trip and hurt herself. If he walked up to her to let her know about the hazard, would she have said, "Get out of my way, sonny. It's none of your beeswax"? Dan had to find out. After approaching her, she replied, "I'm sorry if this looks bad to you, but I have arthritis so bad that I cannot bend over to tie my shoelaces."

Dan kneeled down and asked, "Do you mind if I touch your foot and tie them for you?" This God moment reminded me of the story from the Bible when Jesus actually washed the feet of his twelve disciples. Every week Dan writes down and keeps track of how God's hands are working for us.

One day this man was getting ready to take a cross-country trip through the mountains, but first he had to take his older model car into the shop for service. You see, vandals had broken his antenna, and he just had to have his radio music and talk (Cathy and Judy, the girlfriends) to keep him company. Well, when this man went back to pick up his car, the mechanic shook his head and said, "We did you a great favor, sir. You would have never made it out of the Rocky Mountains if we also hadn't repaired your brakes." God was looking out for that gentleman at the right moment.

And to conclude my sermon, I would like to mention a dream about two sets of footprints in the sand. This faithful parishioner would take long walks in the sand on her favorite beach. When everything was going smoothly, she would notice another set of footprints right next to hers. But on days when she had a hard time coping with life's little surprises, she would not notice that extra set of footprints. She thought that she was all alone when times were hard. But actually the one set of footprints was made by God, carrying the woman in his arms...in her dreams.

So whether you're having a BAKING SODA moment like the kids experienced or a GOD MOMENT that Dan revealed, the gracious Almighty Lord will always be there for you...in good times and also in hard times. Let's pray.

Rocky was in the limelight with his kids that day. He was escorted out of the church by a high-ranking official of the Lord. Pastor Brian concluded, "Since I chose you today to pick on, Rocky, I'll allow you to leave early. Let's boogie."

EPITAPH

Norman 'Rocky' Rauch was born on March 11, 1942—and lost his fight in this world on April 11, 2007 to take the high road. His Lord fulfilled all of his dreams. He raised the bar to live Philippians 4:13 from the Word of God.

www.ingramcontent.com/pod-product-compliance
Lightning Source LLC
Chambersburg PA
CBHW060254290526
45789CB00001B/330